HYPNOSIS
IN CLINICAL PRACTICE

HYPNOSIS
IN CLINICAL PRACTICE

STEPS FOR MASTERING
HYPNOTHERAPY

RICK VOIT, PH.D.
MOLLY DELANEY, PSY.D.

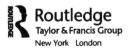
Routledge
Taylor & Francis Group
New York London

Routledge
Taylor & Francis Group
711 Third Avenue
New York, NY 10017

Routledge
Taylor & Francis Group
2 Park Square
Milton Park, Abingdon
Oxon OX14 4RN

© 2004 by Taylor & Francis Group, LLC
Routledge is an imprint of Taylor & Francis Group, an Informa business

First issued in paperback 2013

International Standard Book Number-13: 978-0-415-93544-9 (Hardcover)
International Standard Book Number-13: 978-0-415-86096-3 (Softcover)

Library of Congress Cataloging-in-Publication Data

Voit, Rick.
    Hypnosis in clinical practice : steps for mastering hypnotherapy / Rick Voit, Molly DeLaney.
        p. ;cm.
    Includes bibliographical references and index.
    ISBN 0-415-93544-X
    1. Hypnotism—Therapeutic use. [DNLM: 1. Hypnosis—methods. 2. Physician-Patient Relations.
    WM 415 V898h 2004]   I. Delaney, Molly. II. Title.
    RC495.V615   2004
    616.89'162—dc22   2003017980

Visit the Taylor & Francis Web site at
http://www.taylorandfrancis.com

and the Routledge Web site at
http://www.routledge.com

Contents

Just do the steps that you've been shown
By everyone you've ever known
Until the dance becomes your very own
No matter how close to yours
Another's steps have grown
In the end there is one dance
You'll do alone.

"For A Dancer"
—Jackson Browne

Acknowledgments

The writing of a book such as this is an undertaking that has been touched and influenced by so many people and life experiences that it is difficult to know where to begin. We understand that very few of the ideas expressed in these pages are truly original, as they are based on our exposure to numerous books, professors, supervisors, and, of course, our clients themselves. To all of those who have steered and nudged us toward this work, we offer a heartfelt thank you.

In particular, we wish to express our appreciation to those colleagues who initially brought us together. Included in this group are Frank Rogers-Witte and Julie Linden, who introduced the authors to each other and have since provided invaluable guidance and encouragement. In addition, we must certainly thank Judy Lasher for contributing her energy and enthusiasm as we developed our partnership. We wish to thank John Kasper and those members and faculty of the American Society of Clinical Hypnosis who have provided inspiration, support, and opportunity toward our joint and individual careers. We must certainly acknowledge our Ericksonian friends, particularly Brent Geary and Phil and Norma Barretta, for whom we hold a special fondness and deep gratitude. Brent's interpretation and teaching of hypnotic phenomena have deeply influenced us in our work and our writing. Phil and Norma have become our models for what enduring, collaborative teaching can truly be. We also offer our thanks to the folks at Brunner-Routledge, particularly George Zimmar and Shannon Vargo, for their belief in our project and firm direction toward its completion.

We want to extend a special indebtedness for our friend, colleague, and mentor, Marc Oster, who has nurtured our careers since our first meeting six years ago. No one has had more of an impact on our professional development than Marc. His generous gift of time and constructive criticism as we have prepared our manuscript has been invaluable.

MOLLY

I owe a great debt to my friend and colleague Rick Voit for his courage and enduring persistence in the development of this project. It is likely that our book would never have been completed without his warmth, humor, and tenacity. To my son Max, I extend my deepest appreciation for your encouragement and patience during all those times I was glued to the computer. The same goes for Sweetie, our golden retriever, who missed more than a couple of trips to the park during this process. I give special thanks to my parents, Cormac and Eileen DeLaney, who provided the gift of countless stories proven useful in my teaching and hypnosis. Lastly, my special thanks to the mentors of my early professional days, Milton Erickson, Stephen Gilligan, Erika Fromm, Paul Carter, and David Cheek. Your words and teachings still echo through my work until this day.

RICK

Because I arrived so late on the hypnosis scene, I was not fortunate enough to personally experience the genius of Milton Erickson. I must be content to boast of only "two degrees of separation" from Dr. Erickson through my close association with Dr. DeLaney and the teachings of countless others who shared his company. Instead, I can thank the brilliance of Daniel Brown and his faculty for my early hypnosis education. I owe my comfort and competence in hypnosis to my fellow neophytes, Shelly Plakans, Susanne Pariente, Julie Breskin, and Elizabeth Krafchuk, with whom I shared persistence and enthusiasm that allowed my career to develop as it has. And, of course, I want to thank two early supervisors, Rebecca Shrum and Sam Migdole, for making hypnosis seem so accessible and guiding me toward integrating hypnosis into my practice.

There would be no book without the depth of knowledge and imaginative thinking of my partner, Molly DeLaney. Her associations and stories provide much of the character of this book. Last but not least, I also must thank my dogs, Shamus and Daniel, for constantly reminding me to play on occasion and to not take life all that seriously. We have all survived.

Foreword

It is a pleasure and an honor to write this foreword to Rick Voit and Molly DeLaney's book, *Hypnosis in Clinical Practice: Steps for Mastering Hypnotherapy*. I am especially pleased since I have had the opportunity to observe the evolution of this book from its conception through its development into a completed manuscript. What is gratifying and exciting is that the authors have succeeded in delivering to their readers an accessible and useful manual to enhance practitioners' integration of hypnosis into their work.

While this book might initially appear to be aimed at the novice or intermediate hypnotherapist, its value for all practitioners lies in its excellent suggestions for integrating hypnotic techniques into one's overall clinical orientation and treatment planning. As such, the authors focus more on applied material and admittedly less on didactic material, while assuring the reader that there are ample, excellent sources available and listed in their references. They present their technical information in a clear and precise manner and then, true to their Ericksonian values, make wonderful use of metaphors, as well as personal and clinical stores, to illustrate their message.

Most books about hypnosis practice rarely tell you anything useful about generating hypnosis referrals. *Hypnosis in Clinical Practice* overcomes this flaw by putting into words how to do that which is indicated but seldom well articulated. Specifically, Voit and DeLaney do an excellent job of explaining and showing us how to understand hypnotic phenomena diagnostically and how to use the patient's own talents and behaviors as tools in treatment. Using clinical examples, Voit and DeLaney help clinicians understand how their patients' symptomatic presentation reflects the presence of hypnotic phenomena. By viewing patients in this way, they can better "fit" hypnotic techniques into clinical practice and ultimately facilitate effective treatment planning and the generation of referrals.

Hypnosis in Clinical Practice examines each step in the evolution of the hypnotic relationship and within the hypnotherapist. Among their many examples, Voit and DeLaney each share their stories of their introduction to hypnosis and their development as "hypnotically informed" psychotherapists and how they learned to communicate hypnotically. As I read their story, I recalled my own introduction to hypnotic communication. At the beginning of my hypnosis journey, a fellow workshop participant posed a common question, "What do you do with the person after they are hypnotized?" The instructor offered the following supportive and encouraging replay: "Are you a therapist? (yes) Then you already know what to say once the patient is hypnotized!" He continued, "You are limited only by your lack of creativity." This text emphasizes the origins of a clinician's creativity by directing the reader to investigate the personal and professional roots from which the hypnotic relationship and hypnotic communication grow.

The authors clearly explain that, by removing the mystery of hypnosis for patients, the therapist can demonstrate that the "magic" is the result of their participation in the process. I agree with the authors that this assignment of responsibility and power is critical in overcoming a patient's apprehension and resistance to hypnosis. Such an approach will also facilitate less apprehension about proceeding hypnotically with patients. I often demonstrate glove anesthesia with a new patient for this very purpose. I do it in typical manner that includes my drawing a circle with my finger on the top of their hand while giving the suggestions for the glove anesthesia to manifest. When ready, I take a surgical clamp and ask the patient to watch and tell me what they feel, not what they see, as I pinch a fold of skin on the top of their hand. Their eyes widen as they report no pain, just pressure as I vigorously pinch and pull. When we're finished with the demonstration, I ask again about what they felt, and follow by asking, "And how did you do that?" About half of the patients say they didn't do it, but that I did. In response, I emphasize that I merely drew a circle with my index finger: no magic there. Instead, it is the patients who discover that their ability to turn off the sensation in their hand reveals their own potentials in producing something they deeply desire: the relief of pain. Through this method, they find that the "magic" of hypnosis is within them.

True to their eclectic backgrounds, Voit and DeLaney borrow the Gestalt term "creative indifference" as a means of describing Milton Erickson's openness to all possibilities. In one of the first hypnosis classes I taught at the Adler School of Professional Psychology I gave a demonstration of an arm catalepsy induction. It worked wonderfully. One student inquired how often this technique is successful. I replied that, in my experience, it is 100 percent effective and that it has worked every time I've tried it. I followed that comment with the conclusion that this was the first time I had ever attempted it. Then someone asked the truly important question: "What would you have done if, when you released the arm, it had fallen instead of remaining suspended?" I replied that I would have told the subject that this response, the arm falling, was exactly the response I was seeking. I fully agree with Voit and DeLaney that, when "thinking hypnotically," there are no wrong responses, only wrong, inflexible expectations and a failure to make use of opportunities.

The authors encourage the perspective that, the more clinicians become astute observers of their patients' naturally occurring hypnotic phenomena, the more capable they will become in utilizing these "talents" therapeutically. Furthermore, they tell us how to weave hypnosis into one's personal and professional style by allowing it to become a natural extension of what we do. Instead of asking ourselves if or when we should use hypnosis, Voit and DeLaney suggest we ask, "Why not use hypnosis?" All of our communication becomes hypnotic communication.

Voit and DeLaney have something to say, and the hypnosis community will hear them. As talented and inventive therapists and teachers, they show us the true origins of hypnotic magic and its relation to therapeutic creativity. This book will be a valuable contribution to the teaching of hypnosis, hypnotic communication, and hypnotically informed psychotherapy. It is a pleasure to have shared in their experience.

Marc I. Oster, PsyD, ABPH
President and Fellow, American Society of Clinical Hypnosis
Diplomate, American Board of Psychological Hypnosis
Fellow, American Psychological Association
Professor, Adler School of Professional Psychology

Preface:
A Book for Psychotherapists

In recent years, the popular and professional perception of hypnosis seems to have matured beyond myth and magic to one of genuine interest and broader acceptance. These gains have been achieved despite the perpetuation of long-standing, unfounded fears and misconceptions about hypnosis by tabloid talk shows, films, and stage hypnotists. Those of us trained in hypnosis have become familiar with the many ways in which the induction of hypnotic trance has valuable and impressive applications in medicine, dentistry, psychology, and forensics. It is our hope that these benefits in the enhancement of performance, physical and emotional healing, and everyday functioning have not escaped the attention of the healthcare community and its public in their search for more efficient, less intrusive solutions.

Despite dramatic evidence of the effectiveness of hypnosis and its wider acceptance, only a small percentage of healthcare providers seem to include it in their therapeutic repertoire. In addition, we have often encountered colleagues who have learned basic hypnosis skills but never really introduced them into practice. We believe that this apparent reticence to make greater use of hypnosis may originate from residual misconceptions about the hypnotic process and the potential for failure.

It is the purpose of this book to allay apprehensions about hypnosis by proposing a more realistic and naturalistic view of trance and a less complicated method for the integration of hypnosis into the practitioner's treatment planning. We do not intend to teach specific hypnotic skills or even to substantiate our assertions with an exhaustive review of the literature. Instead, we offer a useful guide for clinicians who wish to seize the opportunities their new skills might create. Our intention is to "fuse" hypnotic technique and a naturalistic view of the hypnosis subject with the existing style and competencies of the psychotherapist. We expect this hypnotic frame of reference regarding human behavior and symptom organization to create a "flow" whereby hypnosis can become a more instinctive extension of one's work. Hopefully, the awkwardness and self-conscious hesitance of the neophyte hypnotherapist will gradually evolve into genuine, assertive confidence.

As evidenced by the apparent large numbers of poorly qualified and laypeople who practice hypnosis, we might conclude that virtually anyone can learn to induce a trance. As our clients adopt self-hypnosis for relaxation and personal growth, they too could likely apply these skills with others. If we agree that trance induction is so easy to learn, what makes its use sometimes so daunting to professionals? Our speculation is that it is their commitment to quality service and positive outcome that creates this apprehension. Ironically, it is this very commitment that should ensure the appropriate and effective use of hypnosis. And, as with any mode of treatment, your "performance" will become more a function of overall clinical expertise than merely the sophistication of hypnotic intervention.

For the most part, practitioners of hypnosis employ similar processes of creating a focused, absorbed state of consciousness in their subjects for the pursuit of appropriate and desirable outcomes within their areas of expertise. Their beginning hypnosis training has likely been similar. As students of hypnosis, they have typically been provided with a history of hypnosis, ethical considerations, and definitions of trance as it occurs naturally and in the clinical setting. Universally useful techniques of induction, deepening, and hypnoprojective suggestion will become the foundation for more advanced applications. While practitioners' skills, styles, and purposes may vary, they all wish to access the unconscious mind and its awesome potentials in order to minimize suffering and provide a relief from physical or psychological symptoms.

It is likely that much of this book would be helpful to any health-care professional wishing to gain greater comfort with her hypnotic skills. However, our focus here will be on the psychotherapist and the ways in which hypnosis and psychological process are so uniquely interrelated. Therefore, we are assuming that the reader works in a mental health setting and that psychological theory and technique are a beginning point for integrating hypnosis into clinical work. Furthermore, we would hope that anyone intending to use hypnosis in the treatment of psychological symptoms has already achieved an advanced level of training and experience in psychotherapeutic theory and practice.

We can assume that hypnosis in the fields of medicine and dentistry is usually dedicated to the treatment of a single symptom, such as pain or anxiety, or to better facilitate healing and recuperation. It is a time-limited, focused intervention to prevent, manage, or eliminate symptoms and their complications. Medical practitioners will most likely pursue further training in the hypnotic treatment of specific patient populations, such as in obstetrics, urology, or oncology.

Long before Western medicine was willing to acknowledge the mind/body continuum, hypnosis had been used to treat physiological diagnoses. Only in the last few decades have we begun to understand the extent to which unconscious mental processes influence physiological states (Pert, 1997) and the corresponding effectiveness of hypnosis in this domain. Moreover, with a growing appreciation for the mind/body continuum, psychogenic and physiogenic domains become more intertwined and the distinction between the two is less clear. Yet, as abstract as the distinction between mind and body symptomatology might sometimes appear, we must remain clear that the training received by medical and mental health practitioners is not. Psychologists who treat chronic pain, irritable bowel syndrome, enuresis, or other physiological symptoms certainly must seek the help of medical professionals in ruling out organic bases for these problems before assuming that their treatment is within their professional responsibility. Medical and dental hypnotists must exercise the same discretion in making diagnostic decisions or pursuing a course of treatment. Clinical applications of hypnosis in psychology and medicine overlap, but they are most certainly not the same.

Thus, in contrast to other professions, we believe the integration of hypnosis into the practice of psychotherapy to be unique. For instance, unlike medical and dental hypnosis, we find that hypnotherapy can often serve as the primary treatment. When the goals of treatment are often exploratory and insight-oriented, desired outcomes are usually much less clear or circumscribed. Psychotherapists might use hypnosis to pursue a shift in unconscious process and a client's overall functioning rather than a single, measurable effect. While the primary intention is still the pursuit of improved well-being and positive effects, the possibilities are no less diverse than our clients themselves. We are open to discovery and an individual's unique adaptations to life's challenging and, at times, brutal truths. Unlike the observable outcomes made possible by the use of hypnosis in dentistry, medicine, or performance, our clients might experience the discomfort of confusion and self-examination on their singular paths to emotional health.

As hypnotherapists, we are called upon to use all our professional, interpersonal skills and knowledge to accurately understand each individual. We know the symptoms we treat to be the psychological results of personal history, cognitive style, filtered perception, and emotional projections. We must anticipate our clients' beliefs about therapy and readiness for change. Clinical hypnosis has the potential to address the full breadth of this domain when incorporated as part of a well-established therapeutic relationship and a comprehensive treatment plan.

As we attempt to identify the ways in which hypnosis naturally integrates with the practice of psychotherapy, we begin to notice how the dynamics involved in hypnosis parallel those of the psychotherapeutic relationship. As psychotherapists, we hope to develop rapport and a trusting, cooperative therapeutic alliance. We make use of all information our clients provide us to gain a more empathic understanding of their subjective experience and their barriers to progress. We work to comprehend our clients' view of the world and to communicate our understanding through accurate empathy and a shared language. We magnify our clients' strengths and establish a treatment plan that will target mutually agreed-upon goals and a resolution to unresolved issues. We seek access to important unconscious material in order to facilitate a greater depth of insight and a unique, corrective experience. Our astute observation of nonverbal communication and idiosyncratic language can offer windows into underlying, rigid belief systems and enduring, immobilizing fears. As you strive to find greater comfort and ease with hypnotic skills, we wish to emphasize that these familiar dynamics and processes are also the foundation of effective hypnotherapy.

To further promote a somewhat artificial divergence in the professional application of hypnosis, consider the way in which a psychotherapist might utilize hypnotic phenomena. As you are likely aware, hypnotic phenomena are those aspects of unconscious functioning that are evident in everyday experience and that are often exaggerated in trance states. Most practitioners of hypnosis will utilize these phenomena for induction, trance ratification, and even therapeutic gains. Yet, many experts in the field of hypnosis (Erickson, Rossi, & Rossi, 1976; Gilligan, 1987; Geary, 2001a) also believe that by diagnosing our clients in terms of the hypnotic phenomena inherent in their behavior, clinicians of any therapeutic discipline can often gain a unique insight into their clients' symptoms, resistances, and means of functioning that other modes of treatment cannot sufficiently provide. The psychotherapist who grasps that hypnotic phenomena are present in everyday, waking-state functioning can best understand how their clients have remained "stuck" in symptoms that they also long to eliminate. And just as important for the clinician practicing hypnosis, attention to the phenomena a client exhibits provides a natural starting point for hypnotherapeutic intervention. We believe such a conceptualization of hypnosis and behavior to be the exclusive domain of psychotherapy.

If the work of therapy and hypnosis is directed by the goals, expectations, and unconscious processes of one's client, it should also be determined by the existing expertise of the therapist. The treatment of emotional and psychological symptoms incorporates unique procedures and processes that should only be undertaken by a professional with sufficient psychological training. As with any ethical and effective psychotherapy, hypnotherapists should only treat conditions for which they are experienced and trained to treat without hypnosis. One must have ample training and supervision to assume competency in treating any diagnostic category with any therapeutic procedure. In other words, if you have never treated eating disorders with traditional psychotherapies, you would not undertake treating them with hypnosis. If you have not worked with children or adolescents in your general practice, you would not pursue hypnosis with these populations either. One tool does not a carpenter make.

It is important to note that the term "hypnotherapy" is itself somewhat controversial. Many believe that hypnosis is not a *therapy* per se, but rather a technique such as a behavioral strategy or a cognitive restructuring intervention. For the purpose of this book, use of the term "hypnotherapy" indicates the use of hypnotic interventions within a psychotherapy setting. We advocate that this text be used by licensed professionals in psychology, social work, psychiatry, nursing, and counseling who practice psychotherapy.

Thus, this book is written with the psychotherapist in mind. More specifically, it is intended to help therapists with prior training in clinical hypnosis to achieve a greater comfort and depth of understanding as they assimilate hypnotic skills into their work. There are many more scholarly and thorough resources available to the beginning and advanced hypnotherapist (Erickson et al., 1976; Gilligan,

1987; Hammond, 1990; Watkins, 1987; Weitzenhoffer, 1989). Our effort
here is to be intentionally straightforward in minimizing confusion
and performance anxiety for the hypnotherapist who might feel awkward in applying hypnotic interventions. At first glance, the reader
might perceive this book to be a rehashing of basic hypnosis training.
In some ways, this would be an accurate assessment. In fact, we are
expecting that our readers will already know much of what we will
be covering in the next eight chapters. There are many elemental skills
that we will not review, but this does not suggest that we believe them
to be unimportant or not helpful. They make up part of the "mechan-
ics" of hypnosis that will eventually become part of your integrated
approach to hypnotic treatment.

Instead, we are hoping to highlight those aspects of hypnosis that
will facilitate its smoother integration into practice. With such "fresh
eyes," much of what you already know will appear more natural and
accessible. In our introduction, we will pay closer attention to the roots
of anxiety that prevent the integration of hypnosis into practice. In
chapter 1, our focus is on how the way you think about hypnosis can
affect your level of comfort with its use. Chapters 2 through 4 establish
a beginning point for hypnotic intervention by encouraging a thorough yet naturalistic framework for a hypnotic relationship. Finally,
chapters 5 through 8 examine an inherent extension of this framework
toward hypnotic induction and treatment.

We simply encourage our readers to imagine themselves sitting
safely and comfortably in the position of a skilled psychotherapist.
From that vantage point, you will allow a perspective on hypnosis to
develop, one that does not change your style or your beliefs about
psychotherapy. It is possible, however, that your view of your clients
and your hypnosis skills might evolve to something excitingly new
and challenging.

Introduction:
The Myth of Magic

The practice of psychotherapy is an inexact blend of science and art that involves complex interpersonal dynamics and, often, uncertain and tenuous outcomes. Clinicians seek out training opportunities to explore and gain mastery of new ideas and strategies in the pursuit of greater success and, of course, a steady flow of referrals. Unfortunately, latent fears of being ineffective may engender self-doubts in the therapist and, consequently, a hesitancy to assert herself creatively within the therapeutic relationship. Considerations regarding one's professional reputation and financial success will limit risk-taking and a willingness to experiment.

Hypnosis seems to produce just such a bind for those who have gained a rudimentary and superficial achievement of hypnosis skills. Psychotherapists who might be initially drawn to hypnosis because of its mystique as a powerful therapeutic tool then become uncomfortable with this same illusion of power. They might expect that a demonstration of these mysterious new phenomena could convince clients of either their newfound effectiveness or their total incompetence. The myth underlying this double-edged sword is that the hypnotherapist, not the client, assumes the responsibility for making therapeutic change possible. The promise of magic must certainly require a skillful magician.

Obviously, a therapist who believes that he holds the reins of his client's hypnotic experience and the client's successful recovery is very likely to fail. This self-induced challenge can be further complicated by the client's corresponding misconceptions, skepticism, and doubts about whether he can "be hypnotized." The potential for a power struggle is clear: The hypnotherapist must prove her power, convince the skeptic, and cure the client in order for the therapy to be considered successful. The resulting anxiety from such unrealistic expectations prevents a more naturalistic approach to using hypnosis and inhibits its broader application. Fears of ineffectiveness and powerlessness will likely tap into any prior conscious or unconscious anxieties the therapist has about using new skills and becoming embarrassed with inadequacy. This self-consciousness will likely contaminate the therapist's responsiveness, objectivity, and even his ability to establish rapport.

Hypnosis is a powerful therapeutic intervention that draws upon the therapist's creativity and spontaneity in a manner that is unmatched by most other interventions. In this way, it is an attractive and exciting alternative. Yet hypnotic phenomena are anything but magical. They make up an integral part of the fabric of our everyday experience. One of the pervasive myths about trance is that it is an atypical way of functioning. Nothing could be further from the truth. Individuals experience trance states and trance phenomena all the time (Erickson & Rossi, 1979). We merely fail to recognize these experiences as "trances" or see them as unusual when they occur in everyday life. Every time we drift off into a daydream, lose track of time, experience that half-awake, half-asleep hypnogogic state between sleep and wakefulness, we are experiencing trance phenomena. Whenever we become deeply absorbed in a book, movie, or intimate conversation we are likely engaging in the kind of focused attention found in trance states. In these situations, we experience a momentary or extended state of trance, where our usual state of reference is briefly disoriented (Rossi, 1996).

These examples of common everyday trance have obvious implications for the practice of hypnotherapy. With trance occurring so naturally and frequently, there is simply no need for a therapist to "do" anything other than to access this talent. Success lies in the recognition and utilization of trance behavior, not in its creation. In reality, a good hypnotherapist is not a magician, but rather an astute observer of human behavior who has learned how to access her clients' inherent hypnotic skills in ways that help them relieve their symptoms. Indeed, the more familiar the therapist becomes with hypnotic phenomena and begins to view her clients in this way, the more likely it is that she will see how these phenomena are inherent in both normal behavior and symptom expression.

To borrow a term from Gestalt psychotherapy, a therapist wants to enter into this relationship with "creative indifference" (Wulf, 1996), maintaining a nonjudgmental openness to all possibilities, internal and external. Milton Erickson made masterful use of this posture. He worked under the premise that whatever the client presented was functional, adaptive, and useful (Zeig, 1980). The "indifference" or neutrality necessary for a successful treatment is nearly impossible if a therapist carries a hidden agenda of monitoring her own performance while also attempting to manage performance anxiety.

An integral theme of this book is that, in all treatment, a therapist's role is to guide her client toward finding his own answers. It is not to bear the full responsibility for a particular outcome or "cure." This is particularly true with hypnosis, where the course of therapy is significantly influenced and even directed by the client's unconscious process and behavior. It is the hypnotherapist's obligation to be prepared and, of course, observant. This simply means that she must be well-grounded and professional in her therapeutic orientation and that she has advanced and integrated her skills in hypnosis so as to be consistent with her orientation.

HYPNOSIS AS A DANCE

Hypnosis could be compared to a dance. Can you imagine dancing with someone who is unconscious, unable to hear the music, uncooperative, or who has no sense of rhythm? You would be completely responsible for the performance, the form, and the grace. It would be a rather awkward, dissatisfying encounter. Instead, hypnosis suggests a sharing of the movement. The hypnotherapist leads: sensing, responding, guiding his partner, who tenses and relaxes along with the leader. The music plays in the background as the therapist and client find a groove, and the client is led into her own dance, movement, and style. Working in this way presupposes that your client, like a dance partner, has the necessary resources to move in the right direction, rather than being an uncoordinated beginner with whom the therapist is responsible for teaching each step.

A perfect example of this dance-like communication is the nonverbal induction. In one version, the "Postural Sway" (Watkins, 1987), the client is encouraged to focus on some nonverbal cue, beginning the communication that will lead him to focus his attention on the therapist. The hypnotist gently touches the client's shoulders as they begin to respond to each other's subtle sway. The client's focus is on this movement and his own internal sensory experience. They dance into trance together, as one (Watkins, 1987). Another version is the handshake induction, in which the hypnotist seems to be merely shaking the subject's hand (Erickson et al., 1976). However, the hypnotist's hand lingers and he alternately releases and applies pressure with his fingers to different parts of the subject's hand. This induces confusion in the subject that is heightened by the therapist focusing not on the subject's face but a bit beyond it. To witness or experience a nonverbal induction offers an appreciation for the redundancy of words and the role of the client's internal cues in establishing trance.

As with all hypnosis, the nonverbal induction is simply a means of establishing communication with the subject's unconscious by leading and responding to her natural movement. Just as you might lead with a dance partner, in hypnosis you can guide the use of your client's innate hypnotic skills to create a therapeutic trance. The dance continues through careful attention to the therapeutic relationship and the opportunities for creativity resulting from this dynamic interaction. Hypnosis, as with any effective psychotherapy, is most powerful when the therapist practices sound clinical procedure and establishes trust and rapport. Educating your client about hypnotic processes removes the mystery of hypnosis while also helping her to see that the "magic" is a result of her cooperation and participation in the therapy process. Once taught the steps, she becomes a willing and graceful dance partner.

SKILL AND STYLE

It will be stressed throughout this work that practicing hypnosis involves both skill and style (Havens, 1985). While scientists seek to establish credibility and standards for this specialty through their rigorous research, we continue to be inspired by the artistry of the masters. Those fortunate enough to have traversed the miles to witness Erickson's charismatic originality were awed not only by his science, but even more so by his artistry. Yet it should not be overlooked that when Erickson was teaching his seminars from his Phoenix home, he already had decades of clinical practice behind him. He was an astute observer of the subtleties of human behavior and used this knowledge like an artful sculptor who hits the marble with his chisel and mallet in such a way as to free huge chunks of unnecessary stone. Such is the work of a therapist: sometimes elegant, sometimes forceful and direct.

Of course, even artists must learn technique at some point. Painters will begin with exercises in color, contrast, and shading in their early education, until their own creativity and self-expression translate skill into something truly unique. Their products will only then become both original and, most likely, technically sophisticated. Like the artist, a hypnotherapist learns basic skills as a broad-brush background. With continued education, supervised practice, sufficient experience, and a grasp of hypnotic communication, she can begin to add the layers of detail that will produce a truly original work of art. Skill comes with repeated practice, while style is developed as the therapist comes to know and develop her inherent talents.

We learn new skills through our training, but our style arises from inside. We urge that as you study and practice hypnosis, you revisit your beliefs about people, life, and relationships and that you become fully aware of what types of work make you confident or anxious. For this reason, we encourage clinicians to become familiar not only with their clients' unconscious processes but their own as well. We would suggest that beginning hypnotherapists will benefit from becoming truly comfortable with the process of hypnosis by seeking personal experience with either heterohypnosis (hypnotherapy between a therapist and client) or autohypnosis (self-hypnosis).

A frequent mistake hypnotherapists make is to attempt techniques with clients that they themselves have not experienced. One of our seminar students once complained that she was unable to elicit trance with her clients using the eye roll technique or hand levitation. However, the therapist herself had never experienced these techniques. Experience is indeed the best teacher. Once therapists become familiar with the "feel" of these techniques themselves, replicating them with their clients becomes much easier. By allowing yourself to listen to your fears and recognize their origins, you can begin to fully utilize a broader range of information in enhancing your therapeutic communication.

For example, while attending a workshop with David Cheek, MD, I (MD) served as a demonstration subject for pain control. Dr. Cheek utilized ideomotor signaling, a technique which I had not yet used either personally or with patients. I was amazed to find my fingers autonomously moving in response to his questions. This experience not only gave me another means to work with my own unconscious but also has become a technique that is invaluable in my work. Continually using hypnosis for your own development can augment your intervention strategies with clients. Not only can it help you to achieve your personal goals, it can also educate you to the variety of experiences you can employ therapeutically with your clients.

Taking such a conscientious approach to the integration of hypnosis into your practice is also helpful in gaining comfort with the skills themselves. A supervisor early in my (RV) hypnosis training reminded me to "think like a therapist." She encouraged me to first and foremost consider what I already knew in assessing my client and to use this foundation to direct my use of hypnosis in her therapy. This advice was both reassuring and encouraging as I began to create more appropriate expectations for what hypnosis was and how it fit into my work.

PATIENCE AND PRACTICE

We urge you to be patient with your development as a hypnotherapist. At the conclusion of his beginning hypnosis training, we overheard a young man excitedly saying, "I'll get my intermediate and advanced trainings out of the way this fall and get certified next winter." While his enthusiasm can be appreciated, his means of becoming a hypnotherapist are obviously naive and even worrisome. He must understand that a psychotherapist must incorporate new skills into his existing expertise, breadth of practice, and personal style. We believe that the practice of psychotherapy and hypnosis in particular are always works in progress.

Whenever we teach beginning hypnotherapists, we strongly encourage them to find ways of practicing their new skills whenever possible. This is the only way they will ever become truly comfortable and effective. There certainly is little practical training available beyond the intermediate level, and it is likely that few successfully pursue ongoing supervision with peers or an approved consultant. For this reason, we have geared our own trainings toward this very population, hoping to revisit the essentials of hypnotherapy in a way that encourages meaningful treatment planning and the development of a style consistent with one's own professional and personal qualities.

The frequent, systematic consideration of hypnosis with each of your clients can help in both demystifying hypnosis and in gaining a greater appreciation for its limitless therapeutic possibilities. We encourage beginning hypnotherapists not to ask, "Should I use hypnosis with this client?" but instead to ask, "Why *not* use hypnosis?" The achievement of greater comfort with hypnotic skills involves their frequent contemplation whether or not they are actually implemented. In addition, to those clients who begin treatment requesting and expecting hypnosis, why not consider all clients to be *potential* hypnotherapy subjects well before the possibility is introduced with them?

Integrating hypnosis into your therapeutic repertoire can also be likened to a ballet student learning to dance on toe. He has already mastered many forms in order to graduate to this difficult and more refined way of dancing. These advanced movements require more precision, balance, and artistry. Initially, the dancer may feel clumsy and frustrated, perhaps evoking dormant uncertainties about his competence. Yet, through repeated practice, he regains his poise. He stands on toe for increasingly longer intervals and then attempts familiar moves with the addition of this new refinement. Eventually, he once again dances with strength and grace, even on toe.

CHAPTER 1

Thinking about Hypnosis

HYPNOSIS: ONE TOOL

George was a middle-aged college professor who sought treatment (RV) for long-standing complaints of depression, irritable bowel syndrome, and a dangerously low body weight. He had previously been seen by numerous traditional and homeopathic physicians and several frustrated psychotherapists, but his symptoms persisted. After his exhausting search for someone to rescue him from his misery, he expressed both desperation and doubt in anyone's capacity to help him. It was clear that his interest in hypnosis was rooted in his wish for an external solution and, perhaps, a magical cure.

George's life was not lacking in conscious emotional conflicts or external stressors. There were plenty. He disclosed feelings of helplessness due to geographical distance from his aging parents and his inability to help them. Marital communication was suffering and sexual intimacy was nearly nonexistent because of his frail physical condition. He had recently accepted responsibility for a research project that would create even greater demands on his time and energy. Perhaps his greatest stressor was also his greatest need: food. During his youth, he had learned that food was his mother's currency in controlling the

1

family and, by refusing to eat, his means of passive-aggressively controlling her. He was now controlled by rigid beliefs about what he
could eat and was unable to tolerate even normal digestive sensation
(e.g., indigestion, bloating, etc.).

Our treatment plan would need to incorporate manageable goal
setting and waking-state cognitive restructuring to assist him in
achieving success with less self-doubt. I introduced George to hypnosis
with the intent of helping him to control his gastrointestinal discom-
forts, to access his existing ego strengths, and, hopefully, to uncover
any additional unconscious conflicts that might be creating barriers to
improvement.

As his insight grew, his confidence and hope returned as well. We
established reasonable goals for helping his parents, communicating
with his wife, and organizing his life. He kept a food diary to avoid
dissociation from physical hunger and learned self-hypnosis to therapeutically utilize this "talent" for dissociation to relieve pain. Our
premise was to replace the helplessness of an external locus of control
by establishing personal responsibility for his symptoms. The introduction of hypnosis was but one of several means of achieving this.
Otherwise, his was a comprehensive, multimodal treatment plan
involving cognitive restructuring, behavioral goal setting, and a psychodynamic interpretation of the family system. Yes, the use of hypnosis
enhanced all of these interventions, but it was not the entire treatment.
George has gained weight, continues to journal, works assertively with
his wife toward a better marriage, and uses self-hypnosis for digestion
and pain management. My client was my project, my treatment plan
was my design, and hypnosis was but one tool.

An effective therapist might be compared to a seasoned carpenter,
a craftsman who is skilled in the use of many tools to build or make
repairs. Perhaps the comparison could also be to an artist who uses
various brushes to create texture or light in each unique piece of work.
It is not the saw that makes a cabinet any more than it is the brush
that paints the masterpiece. Rather, it is the creativity and vision of
the hands holding these tools. In this way, hypnosis is a tool or brush,
albeit a potentially powerful one, in the therapist's repertoire.

Friends and acquaintances will often ask us, "What types of clients
do you treat with hypnosis and how does it help?" Despite our years
of training and experience, we find these simple questions difficult to
answer. The most accurate and honest response we could offer would
be, "We don't treat people with hypnosis, we treat them with psychotherapy. Sometimes we use hypnosis as a part of that treatment."

Ironically, the more competent and comfortable with hypnosis we have become, the less we consider these interventions to be a distinct mode of treatment. As we sit with our clients and ponder ways in which we can be helpful, it will suddenly become clear to us that hypnosis is our preferred means to accomplish our objectives. Just as the artist would almost instinctively reach for one of her brushes, the psychotherapist introduces hypnosis at appropriate junctures in treatment. As we practice safely within the bounds of our strengths and specialties, the "reach" for hypnosis becomes a logical and fluid extension of our overall treatment strategy.

Hypnosis and Therapeutic Orientation

Who hasn't lain on a beach or in a field and imagined what the passing clouds might resemble? The images we attribute to these clouds are creative projections of ourselves. We might also describe the beach experience itself in terms that reflect our memories or sensory strengths. An otherwise universal experience is influenced by our individuality. Not only do we tend to prefer a particular sensory system, but also no two individuals will see, feel, or hear a shared experience identically. Like our fingerprints, our projections and the way we receive information are unique to each of us.

It is likely that any of our clients and their symptoms would be described quite differently by various therapists depending on their clinical belief systems and their personal experiences. A psychodynamic therapist would certainly have focused upon George's family history and unresolved developmental conflicts. The behavioral therapist might ostensibly disregard those issues while placing more emphasis on changing eating habits and learning a healthier lifestyle. Whatever your therapeutic frame of reference — psychodynamic, humanistic, behavioral, etc. — you conceive of humans and their strengths and challenges in a certain way. This frame of reference becomes the basis for a treatment plan that reflects your own clinical interpretations, thus allowing you greater comfort and confidence with the hypnotic applications.

While you maintain your preferred orientation, hypnosis will become a new tool in your toolbox. You are not required to think or even behave in a new way. You simply must work from your roots, with a solid understanding of your professional limits. You are not expected to change, only grow.

As you read the story of George, no doubt you were forming your own ideas as to how you might have approached his symptoms. In my work with him, hypnosis was utilized toward several goals, including insight development, ego strengthening, and behavioral change. Additionally, the increasingly obvious benefits of its use facilitated greater trust and positive transference from my client. The essential point is that, regardless of your frame of reference, hypnosis can provide a valuable ingredient to your treatment plan while facilitating a more fluid conception and implementation of that plan. It might be helpful to briefly examine a few theoretical orientations and identify how hypnosis might come into use.

As a *psychodynamic* therapist, you might use hypnosis to correct neurotic patterns of behavior that began in childhood but are no longer "necessary" as an adult. Making use of hypnotic projections and recovered memories, a client might realize a long-awaited corrective experience that can allow for a healthier definition of himself.

For example, one client (MD) recovered through hypnosis a childhood of petting and playing with baby chicks in her backyard as her mother hung laundry on a clothesline. She recalled becoming distressed when one of the chicks stopped moving. Her mother quickly realized the chick had died, commenting, "I guess you loved it too much." This offhanded, accidental empathic failure apparently contributed to the client's belief that her affections were dangerous. Although this incident had not been the foundation for all of her fears and guilt associated with being playful or intimate, the recovery of this particular memory was significant. It helped her to realize where some of her long-standing barriers to love and self-esteem had developed. Traditional psychoanalytic therapy without hypnosis would likely have taken much longer to reach such a breakthrough.

A *cognitive* therapist might use hypnosis to help her client more easily integrate new and more constructive ways of thinking and behaving toward life's encounters and demands. Rigid, ineffective belief systems are deeply integrated into perception and are possibly more readily accessed with hypnotic communication with the unconscious. Much of our thinking, our belief system "filter," operates unconsciously as we interpret the world into feelings and actions. For example, one gentleman (MD) who was hypersensitive to criticism in his primary relationships with women was able to identify the introjections of his mother's negativity and, instead, create a greater awareness of his achievements and strengths. While typical cognitive therapy is itself considered a "brief therapy," it also requires consistent, frequent challenging of these beliefs in order to interrupt and alter their effect. Hypnosis can more efficiently identify and replace irrational, self-destructive thinking.

A *humanistic* therapist might use hypnosis to help a client more easily recognize his intrinsic goodness and thus enhance his overall functioning. The trusting intimacy of the hypnotic relationship itself can be validating and comforting in the communication of compassion and acceptance. Even our own nurturing voices and positive attitudes encourage hope and well-being. In treating low self-esteem, we might use a positive affect bridge to recover the experience of success from earlier achievements. We believe that every hypnotic intervention should include ego-strengthening affirmations, a hallmark of humanistic approaches.

Marjorie, a hospice nurse, remained in an abusive marriage, believing that this was her lot in life. It wasn't until she was diagnosed with a life-threatening disease that she sought treatment (MD). Her history was replete with instances of abuse, both emotional and sexual, as well as the concomitant shame experiences. By using a combination of ego strengthening, cognitive restructuring, and the integration of her own words into hypnosis, the client began to assert her own desires and aspirations as well as believe she was worthy of achieving these dreams. She had become mobilized to battle her illness as well as to become more assertive in her marriage. When it became obvious to her that her husband had no desire to preserve their relationship, she sought freedom from her marriage. Now, several years later, she believes that therapy saved her life.

A *behavioral* therapist could include hypnosis in treatment in order to build confidence, identify resistance, or clarify goals toward behavior change. For example, in the treatment for smoking cessation, post-hypnotic messages that promote health, healing, and ego strength might be introduced to the unconscious. The therapist can suggest cues or attachments in her client's environment to reduce craving or reinforce a learned response to predictable internal or external events. Internal cues such as cravings for nicotine could be paired with a wish to deeply breathe in fresh air. Each of these deep breaths could be paired with a renewed sense of commitment to the client's goal of being free and feeling proud of his decision. The external cue of seeing other people smoke could be paired with a sense of relief that he is no longer a victim of this deadly habit.

As therapists, our effectiveness would be severely limited if we were to maintain a narrow clinical orientation regardless of the diversity of people we treat. In fact, as our careers progress, we find it increasingly difficult to identify or label exactly what our "approach" might be. It has been our experience that, however well hypnosis can be effectively integrated into an orientation, it also offers an opportunity for creativity and unique options while remaining loosely within that orientation.

I (RV) recently consulted with a colleague who was treating a child afflicted with facial tics. Consistent with her family systems orientation, this psychologist viewed this symptom as a reflection of developmental conflicts, enabling the child to receive attention from doting but emotionally unavailable parents. I introduced the notion that the tic was also dissociative and regressive in nature (both hypnotic phenomena). Her treatment plan will now include an effort to "associate" this girl with her symptom and find healthier means of expressing and managing her conflicts. While hypnosis broadens its scope, the orientation can remain the same.

Accessing All Resources

Because you are likely drawn to a certain theoretical orientation because it makes some kind of personal sense, it might be beneficial to have a firm grasp of the personal and historical elements to your clinical style. Developing insight into your values, beliefs, and biases can prevent you from projecting them intrusively into any treatment approach. Discovering your strengths, weaknesses, and blind spots will only make your hypnotic work richer. Awareness of where your talents begin and end allows for a more seamless and ethical integration of hypnosis into your therapeutic repertoire.

As with the practice of all psychotherapy, integrating hypnosis into your work becomes a product of all you are and all you know. In this regard, it is important to view your personal life experiences, your interests and passions as a rich mine from which you can uncover new and creative initiatives. You probably intuitively draw on your associations, images, remembrances, and thoughts in your present clinical work. In the practice of hypnosis, these are especially helpful resources, as so many of our own associations spring to mind during our unconscious connection with clients. Just about every clinician can tell you of the times when they felt totally in sync with their clients. Associations flow and the resulting interventions are rich and spontaneous. We have found that these occurrences become even more frequent with the use of hypnosis, as you are likely connecting more intimately with your own as well as your client's unconscious processes.

In all of our work, we depend heavily upon our own experiences, how we feel in our own skin. Thus, it is extremely useful to study as a "scientist" our own trance experiences. For example, if you accept the premise that trance is a naturally occurring event that is universally experienced, you should be able to ascertain when your own trance behaviors take place. Indeed, if consciousness is a wavelike pattern (Rossi, 1993), you should be able to become aware of those varying experiences within yourself. It is likely that many of those moments you have heretofore identified as "fatigue" are rather the door opening to your own spontaneous trance. Can you likewise take these moments as an opportunity to go into trance and allow yourself to reenergize? Having done so, can you identify the impact of utilizing these spontaneous trances?

It is important for the therapist to become intimately familiar with his own trance experience. In many ways, insights gained from being the hypnotic subject can provide the raw material from which we build our empathic hypnotic connection with clients. For example, I (MD) used hypnosis while undergoing treatment for a medical condition that required several surgeries. As is common with surgical clients, the use of hypnosis not only alleviated my anxieties about the procedures, but also minimized my need for pharmacological anesthesia and lessened my recovery time. In fact, with my last outpatient surgery, the medical staff was astounded when I was ready to be discharged an hour after awakening from anesthesia. Hypnosis significantly relieved my experience with surgery, while subsequently influencing my pre-surgical work with clients. By experiencing firsthand the tremendous help hypnosis could be for me, I became impressed with its potential benefits for others. I often relate these types of experiences to clients both in and out of hypnosis as a form of suggestion, a metaphor to indicate the possibilities they can as well achieve with hypnosis.

As a scientist it is important for you to study both your clients and yourself as the principal ingredients in creating effective psychotherapy. Whether you notice it or not, your clients are spontaneously experiencing trance during your sessions. Trance behavior may be elicited by their biological need to experience a daydream, or it may be evoked by the work that is taking place in the session. In either case, it is a moment in time that is replete with possibilities.

As the artist, you can create suggestions or metaphors that will be received with little conscious resistance. By becoming attuned to your client's and your own natural rhythms you create opportunities for rapid intervention that could otherwise be missed. Unfortunately, therapists sometimes view their client's "inattention" as boredom or resistance when in fact it has been the client being absorbed in a trance experience triggered by the therapy.

Likewise, by deliberately evoking your own trance, you can not only minimize the tendency so many therapists have toward succumbing to "empathic fatigue," but also facilitate the growth of your hypnotherapy skills. Personal experience with our own trance phenomena teaches us much about the potentials of hypnosis beyond what we learn by simply performing our skills.

Imagine Cro-Magnon man who is considered to have possibly been the first to create art. These ancestors apparently had a wish to leave permanent renderings of what they saw and, perhaps, how they felt. There were no finished tools or brushes to buy or prior creation from which to learn. Instead, they utilized what they had. Their imagination provided inspiration, pigmented earth and perhaps animal blood were their media, and crude instruments and their hands were their only tools. Having little else with which to work, they used the very fabric of their lives in leaving their mark on unwritten history.

A career in hypnotherapy is painted in much the same way. Our personal histories and interpersonal styles create the background. Our clinical training determines the subject of our work as we emulate the innovations of our mentors. We then add detail using whichever methods and tools we have learned to favor. Finally, we discover that hypnosis can bring a greater depth of color and texture to our work. We are not changing a thing about ourselves, our visions, or our styles. All of these influences continue to contribute as they previously had. Rather, we have added one tool, one very helpful and effective tool, in completing each and every masterpiece.

The Role of Hypnosis

To further underscore the suggestion that hypnosis is but a therapeutic tool and not a treatment approach per se, we remind the reader that hypnosis can be either the central focus of therapy or an adjunct to other modes of treatment. As a major intervention in therapy, hypnotherapy can paint a new, more hopeful background for life in the foreground. It can rebuild an old, tattered ego structure into a more secure and functional existence. Hypnosis can be a dramatic method for helping our clients to move forward with their lives, often with less resistance and psychological pain than is common in more waking-state therapies. We can reconstruct belief systems, redefine memories, and establish new confidence (Erickson et al., 1978; Gilligan, 1987; Yapko, 2003). We can help the client to experience a greater sense of efficacy and empowerment with an improved sense of entitlement and confidence. As an adjunct to treatment, hypnosis might be used to help the client develop health-promoting relaxation skills, manage physical or emotional pain, improve performance, or encourage the unconscious to work between sessions of a waking-state mode of treatment (Hammond, 1990). In George's case, hypnosis became both the primary intervention for ego reconstruction as well as a means of treating specific symptoms. As a broad brushstroke, I helped him to develop a more functional self-image while also addressing the "detail" of physical experience and daily functioning. With our therapeutic relationship as the canvas, we used all tools, all brushes, to achieve a successful and satisfying outcome.

All that being said, we offer one very important caveat. You will occasionally be asked to see other therapists' clients for smoking cessation, performance anxiety, or pain management interventions while the core of psychotherapy is to remain the domain of your referring colleagues. Considering that hypnosis is practiced by medical professionals in just such an isolated format, an adjunct role for a psychotherapist could certainly work without any difficulty. However, as you likely already know, we never know the full complexity of a presenting symptom until we actually encounter its sufferer. I (RV) recall one particular client who was referred by a practice partner. My colleague had expressed the opinion that his treatment of this man for a dysfunctional family history was nearly complete and that I was being asked to help with fibromyalgia pain management. Upon meeting this man, I discovered how little progress he had made in his psychotherapy and, more importantly, how "functional" his symptoms were as they intertwined with his family dynamics. Yes, he would benefit from hypnosis, but only if it were in the context of what I knew to be his greater need for a comprehensive treatment plan.

Thus, we strongly suggest that, before you agree to treat someone else's client with hypnosis, you first meet with him at least once to determine how clearly your role can be defined. Otherwise, the potential for actually contributing to your client's problems could be significant.

CONCEPTUALIZING HYPNOSIS: BEYOND DEFINITIONS

How Do We Define Trance?

At this point, we have established that hypnosis is a collection or sequence of skills that facilitates a unique process toward the creation of a therapeutic trance. Those skills can be written, taught, learned, and practiced by almost anyone, hopefully a trained and licensed professional. Yet how do we even begin to interpret the phenomena referred to as trance? We can measure heart rate (Watkins, 1987) and skin temperature (Watkins, 1987) and call it "trance," but the experience is so very subjective and personal that it is nearly impossible to isolate descriptors that are consistent from one subject to another. One client (RV) reported she was uncomfortable with the idea of being hypnotized, preferring to label her trance state as "my peace." This word somehow reflected an element to trance that felt consistent with her experience while also maintaining her need for control.

Most hypnosis texts eventually attempt to formulate a definition of trance. Despite years of research and practice, the debate continues as to just what happens when we hypnotize our clients. Some believe that trance is an altered state of mind, as the conscious and unconscious "dissociate" or split. The conscious mind is occupied and absorbed in one thing, while the unconscious mind is off doing something else (Weitzenhoffer, 1989).

Others believe that trance is more a state of heightened suggestibility created by the hypnotic relationship; one person is trusting, expecting, and willing to be influenced by the suggestions of another (Weitzenhoffer, 1989; Erickson et al., 1976; Gilligan, 1987). The therapist and client enter into a shared experience where they utilize the client's readiness to explore new, creative opportunities in order to facilitate healing or conflict resolution.

We are choosing not to continue this debate here. For the purpose of helping the reader to become a competent, confident hypnotherapist, we are viewing trance as both: an altered state of consciousness that is a process rather than an outcome. We access in our clients their natural talent to achieve a trance state through which they are influenced by our therapeutic suggestions.

However it may be defined, it appears that entering into trance is a naturalistic phenomenon that we all have the capacity to do. Trances occur effortlessly and spontaneously. Some experts believe that we go into trance in a cycle similar to dream states during sleep. It is believed that we have a wave pattern of alertness and daydreaming that typically runs for approximately one and one-half to two hours (Rossi, 1993, 1996). Citing research begun in the 19th century by the French neurologist Jean-Martin Charcot, Ernest Rossi writes: "Another century of research was required before laboratory scientists coined the term *ultradian* and recognized that our nighttime dreams take place every 90 to 120 minutes when we sleep, while our daydreams follow the same rhythm when we are awake" (Rossi, 1996). We think of it as the mind/body's way of "recharging the batteries." Not unlike dream states, we "go internal" whether we are aware of it or not.

We are already familiar with "highway hypnosis," where the conscious mind is occupied with random thoughts or attention to the radio. The unconscious mind does quite well in safely driving toward an expected destination. We would suggest to parents that, when their child is engrossed in a video game and doesn't respond to their comments, he is not necessarily being oppositional. He is demonstrating the product of a natural, dissociative state coupled with an enjoyable activity. Going in and out of trance is, therefore, quite common, natural, and often entertaining. If we accept this premise that trance is a naturally occurring state of consciousness, then we understand that the responsibility for attaining that experience belongs to your client. Furthermore, understanding who owns this responsibility serves to reduce therapist performance anxiety and to empower your client with a potent access to valuable material.

From the moment you shift the responsibility for trance to your client, you have essentially begun to introduce self-hypnosis and its potentials for relaxation, memory access, and symptom relief. As you guide her through her innate talents, you are implicitly expressing a belief in her capacity to enter trance and to use it for improvement. With your induction, you are reinforcing the naturalistic qualities of trance and, through your hypnotic interventions, you are demonstrating the power of the unconscious and how this power is readily available for symptom management. By placing the trance experience more consciously and unconsciously in your clients' grasp, you provide them with the choice of mastering dysfunctional learning that may have occurred during periods of earlier life suggestibility.

While we are not intending to offer our readers a method for teaching clients self-hypnosis, we encourage you to do so. We simply wish to emphasize the following sequence of ideas. Hypnotherapists can minimize performance anxiety by understanding the true nature of trance and the client's natural abilities to enter trance. In performing hypnosis, we access those abilities and utilize them in treatment. Our clients are simultaneously learning to recognize unconscious processes that had not been a part of their conscious, focused awareness. Once enlightened, clients may begin to enter a trace independently of the external induction process and to exploit their newly discovered talents for self-hypnosis.

Thus, trance becomes redefined for the hypnotherapist and the client. The responsibility and empowerment is now "owned" by the client, and, in the process, conscious resistance and apprehension are minimized and the hypnotherapist can behave more freely and creatively.

Unconscious Process in Psychopathology

People suffering from anxiety and depression spend much of their lives in trance (Gilligan, 1987). Such clients could be conceptualized as being stuck in a dysfunctional trance state. If we are viewing trance as a focused, absorbed state of consciousness, then we can appreciate how depression involves a total immersion in negative thinking, physical lifelessness, and overwhelming emotions. Imagine the depressed person, shoulders slumped, often seemingly unable to raise his head or eyes, his thought patterns in a similar rut of demeaning or hopeless dialogue. His detachment from life is obvious, as he goes around and around in an endless cycle of pain. The anxious client is likewise "stuck." Unable to manage her racing thoughts and physiological symptoms ranging from stomach disorders to migraines, she continually seeks more control over those symptoms.

In simplistic terms, we might view human behavior as driven by conscious intent but often steered by unconscious motivation and idiosyncratic learning. However desperate people are to escape their symptoms and patterns, they are often prevented from moving forward by an irrational but earnest unconscious effort to do otherwise. The depressed man who struggles to escape his emotional catalepsy could be thwarted by a greater need to escape further pain.

We are often cognitively governed by deeply ingrained learning sets from earlier periods of our lives that still serve as the basis of our responses to life. These learning sets can be considered post-hypnotic suggestions made on impressionable minds at an earlier time. Our unconscious beliefs alter later readings of external stimuli to fit an internal interpretation of the world. In this way, they provide a "filter" through which our perceptions are interpreted and used to alter our view of life. Dysfunctional learning can be viewed as entrenched hypnotic suggestions that have outlived their usefulness and accuracy. The child of an unhappy marriage might act out his anxieties with opposition and defiance. Should these behaviors be punished or labeled as the child's fault, he might grow up with feelings of helplessness and inadequacy. Further experiences with rejection and criticism will reinforce this negative self-image without the benefit of insight. Certainly George *wanted* to eat normally, but his unconscious perpetuated a misguided and unhealthy assertion of control. As with George, hypnosis can help the adult revisit and redefine his past and perhaps relieve himself of unnecessary fear and anger.

As irrational as some beliefs and behaviors may appear to the untrained eye, they have a logic that is somehow functional and ego-syntonic for that person. In this way, symptoms may be viewed as merely variations on the theme of an earlier adaptation. Often the key to helping our clients to identify and achieve necessary change lies in discovering that logic. It is only within the last decade that we have begun to appreciate the impact that trauma has on a human organism (van der Kolk, McFarlane, & Weisaeth, 1996). Traumatic events can be something as dramatic as a significant or sudden loss, being sexually abused, or witnessing violence, or something as subtle as the criticism of a teacher or parent at just the "right moment." That is, the ordeal occurred at a time or age, when, for whatever reason, the person was highly suggestible. This is not to imply that there are not biological bases for mental illness, rather that there is a combination effect. Poor boundaries, impaired mental functioning, and/or chaotic emotional states that are the result of faulty biology leave the client more susceptible to the impact of others or the environment. Retreating into symptomatology such as dissociation, paranoia, depression, or anxiety are ironically attempts to make the world safe. On an unconscious level, it makes perfect sense for the afflicted client to remain in a dysfunctional trance state.

For example, Caroline presented for treatment (MD) when she developed a fear of riding in elevators. When her employment required that she ride them frequently, this symptom became particularly bothersome. A review of her history revealed that she had become symptomatic following the death of her mother. Although her conscious recollection of childhood had been unremarkable, hypnosis enabled her to recall a significant memory. At the age of 10, she was invited to accompany a friend's family on their summer vacation. Caroline's parents discouraged her from going by suggesting that there might be a fire and she could be trapped inside the cottage. She had since repressed the fearful images that their concern had created. It wasn't until she became an adult and her mother was no longer present to "protect" her that she became symptomatic. Thus, her unconscious perpetuated a symptom it "believed" to be protective and necessary. By understanding the origin of her fear of enclosed places and controlling her anxiety symptoms with self-hypnosis, Caroline learned to use elevators without fear.

We wish to promote the view that symptoms not only serve a purpose but also create opportunities for hypnotic intervention. In the next chapter, we will review *hypnotic phenomena* and how they are manifested in normal and pathological human behavior. We maintain that a firm understanding of these phenomena will provide you with a view to a diagnostic profile of your clients that facilitates a more natural induction and hypnotic treatment planning. Such a framework will allow you to access trance and not believe you must create it. Furthermore, with an accurate assessment of your clients' existing hypnotic characteristics, the road to healing can become a logical extension of the symptoms themselves.

If dreams are the royal road to the unconscious, hypnosis is the driveway leading to the castle; hopefully, a shorter and more direct route than other methods used in traditional talk therapy. With hypnosis, the therapist can assist her client in approaching difficulties with "new eyes" while accessing internal resources (learning, memories, forgotten feelings) more easily and with less resistance. We see utilizing hypnosis with your clients as a means of helping them to discover a gift they have always had and have already been using unconsciously. The discovery of this gift puts its power more directly in their hands to use for their continued health and happiness.

ETHICAL HYPNOSIS IS EFFECTIVE HYPNOSIS

Frankly, a discussion on the subject of ethics in the practice of psychotherapy can often be received with nervous apprehension, polite disinterest, or outright boredom. Many therapists believe that because they are compassionate, professional caregivers, they are implicitly ethical and capable of determining their own standards and practices. Much of what we do as therapists receives the scrutiny of no one but our clients, who have few informed expectations about the limits of professional behavior. We work in solitude, vulnerable to the potential for misuse of power and influence our position carries with it.

Many of us are perhaps only concerned about how we must behave in our practices to avoid liability and malpractice. In this age of rampant litigation and managed care's intrusiveness into client confidentiality, therapists seem to talk more about record-keeping and billing than quality and effectiveness of care. In this way, the prospect of hearing about ethics is likely to feel like a lecture on how to stay out of trouble rather than on fulfilling the need to better serve our clients.

We, however, take a different view on the subject. It is our opinion that, while ethical guidelines might be primarily intended to protect the public, the profession, and the professional from legal problems, they also limit our work to what we truly know how to do. Like parents imposing logical or natural consequences, our licensing boards and organizations hold us responsible for our actions and teach us to be conscientious. By adhering to these limits, we know that we and our clients are relatively safe from harm and that our work will be, at the very least, competent.

Ethical principles for the use of hypnosis would also provide such protective limitations through which the therapist can feel secure in his actions. He treats clients whom he is fully trained and prepared to treat. He applies theories and techniques only as an extension of his accustomed style and expertise. He will therefore avoid complications to which he is unprepared to respond effectively. He can use all of his skills, including hypnosis, confidently believing that his efforts will be as effective as his talents will allow. In this way, we suggest that the practice of hypnosis within the ethical principles of our disciplines can help to implicitly reduce the hypnotherapist's apprehensions and, as a result, encourage its utilization and integration.

Codes of Ethics

The underlying assumption for this discussion is that our readers are familiar with and routinely practice within the general ethical expectations of their professional organizations. As we have stated, such a rigid observance will itself ensure the competent integration of any new skill.

On the subject of hypnosis, the American Psychological Association (APA) Ethical Principles of Psychologists and Code of Conducts speaks in terms of "integrity," "competence," "professional and scientific responsibility," and "respect for people's rights and dignity," all necessary and worthwhile characteristics for a therapist to possess (2003). The spirit of these words does reflect the position from which we make our assertions regarding ethical and effective hypnosis.

In general, however, we find the tone of the APA Code to be more cautionary than encouraging. While it suggests that its "preamble and general principles are aspirational goals to guide psychologists," it also speaks in terms of "enforcement" and procedures for "resolving complaints of unethical conduct" (American Psychological Association, 2003). Certainly, it is the burden and responsibility of such a major governing body to establish concise professional standards and to hold its constituents accountable to those standards. Yet the ethical standards supported by the APA make few specific recommendations on the topic of hypnosis other than discouraging its practice by laypersons.

The Society for Clinical and Experimental Hypnosis (SCEH) promotes four primary standards for the use of hypnosis: (1) that the hypnotherapist be in good standing with his professional organization; (2) that use of hypnosis be restricted to one's existing area of expertise; (3) that the use of hypnosis be only for purposes of improving health and not be used for entertainment; that hypnosis not be performed by nonprofessionals; and that when advertising hypnosis to the public, that the advertising be responsible and accurate; (4) that hypnosis be used to contribute to the welfare of the patient or research subject (2001). Again, these tenets are simple, straightforward, and essentially mirror those of any responsible professional organization.

The most clear-cut code of conduct pertaining to the use of hypnosis in practice is that offered by the American Society of Clinical Hypnosis (ASCH), and ostensibly echoes the substance and intent of the SCEH Code. Yet, while the ASCH Code (2003) is just as broadly applicable and concise, it is somewhat more specific in a few areas. It adds that when presenting hypnosis to the public, prospective employers, and clients, the clinician should "refrain from unsubstantiated statements." These guidelines are appropriately conservative and make common sense. (See Appendix D.)

Hypnosis workshops conducted by professional organizations such as ASCH and SCEH commonly include a section on the ethics involved in using hypnosis in clinical practice. Like reading the potential side effects of a prescription, the admonitions inherent in these instructions can be daunting and even discouraging. Yet therapists need to remember that whatever therapeutic approach is being used, they need to be guided by common sense and solid clinical practice. It is nearly impossible to establish a set of guidelines to cover all possible uses or abuses of hypnosis. The integrity and professionalism of the practitioner are at the root of independent practice regardless of the specific recommendations of that person's discipline.

The Ethical Practice

It may seem paradoxical that we are advocating that the integration of hypnosis into one's practice is both uncomplicated and ethically fraught with danger. The risks lie primarily in the misuse of hypnosis and/or a failed therapeutic relationship. By attending to the principles you have found effective in your clinical practice and the ethical expectations outlined by major professional hypnosis organizations, you should have both a firm grasp of what ethical hypnosis involves and the ability to naturally develop a more relaxed and positive attitude toward its practice. Ethical work contributes to good work. The more we monitor ourselves to practice hypnotherapy that maintains healthy boundaries, respects the integrity of each client, and is well planned and executed, the more effective we will be.

A Solid Therapeutic Foundation

As we begin our careers as psychotherapists, those theories and techniques that work and feel right for us become integrated, while other ideas are cast aside. Our clinical styles can be further defined by the work settings we enter. I (RV) left graduate school with an interest in pursuing a career as a Gestalt therapist. However, my first position working with a deinstitutionalized, "chronic" population proved to be unsuitable for such emotionally evocative work. My clinical style thus became more pragmatic and solution-oriented as it was redirected more by necessity than interest. Many therapists experience the same serendipity regarding the development of their therapeutic interests and subsequent career paths. Perhaps you have come to this interest in hypnosis in a similar way.

Following graduate school and internships, there are increasingly fewer opportunities to thoroughly learn and adopt new ideas. Most of us have pursued training in hypnosis after completing graduate school, and the availability of adequate supervision in its use and application can be limited. Introductory training in hypnosis usually leaves us able to induce a trance and even evoke a range of hypnotic phenomena; yet, at this stage, we really know very little about the process. The fear of being ineffective and a wish for professional integrity inhibit many of us from doing any work that feels new, unfamiliar, or uncomfortable. There is therapy and then there is hypnosis. They seem related but not yet parts of the same whole.

By definition, in order to integrate any new skill into practice, you must find a way to weave it into something else. That "something else" involves all that you know as a therapist, your personal and professional styles of relating to others, and the characteristics of the clients whom you treat. It is not unlike the beginning of any relationship, where two people learn of each other's similarities and differences and gradually bend and adapt to form a working partnership. Hypnosis will fit immediately into your practice in some ways. In others, there will be a period of altering both your style and hypnotic techniques toward a fusion that works.

Following my initial hypnosis training, I (RV) sought to facilitate this integration by pursuing peer supervision with other relatively novice hypnotherapists. We practiced inductions, discussed our clients, and exchanged information about further training opportunities. By attending numerous conferences given by local and national organizations, I began to consider more difficult clients as possible hypnotic subjects and pursued individual supervision to ensure the effective use of hypnosis in those areas. Until recently, I continued with regular group supervision that has allowed me to refine my skills and discuss therapeutic issues and professional growth. These pursuits have allowed me to establish a greater depth of understanding and level of comfort with a tool that has otherwise seemed to "fit" into my style from the beginning.

In contrast, I (MD) continued my hypnosis training by attending several "intensives" which were held over a period of several days to a week. These smaller, Ericksonian workshops typically included didactic elements, case conferencing, and experiential work that contributed to my developing an individualized approach to hypnotic treatment. I concurrently underwent psychoanalysis and attended a doctoral program that focused upon analytic and family therapy. All of this proved to be quite the smorgasbord of therapeutic approaches to somehow integrate. On several occasions, I would return to school from a week of intensive Ericksonian hypnosis training and suddenly realize how this new knowledge contrasted with my graduate school education. I couldn't help but feel more than a little confused as I tried to figure out how to fit these various parts into a cohesive whole. Eventually, I began to discover how these different ways of thinking complement each other. For example, all three of these schools — psychoanalysis, family systems, and hypnosis — view symptoms as meaningful attempts to address psychological issues. This practice of framing symptoms as a client's unconscious resolution of a dilemma continues to be fundamental to my work.

During a recent workshop on hypnotic treatment planning, we noticed that our beginners were appearing more than a little over-whelmed by all their new knowledge. They seemed tired and almost shell-shocked. One student groaned, "I feel like I've had too much to eat." In an effort to frame their predicament in metaphoric terms, we asked if they had ever filled a jar with something, maybe coffee beans, only to have a little left over. If they gently shook the container, its contents could settle and make room for the rest of the beans. We expressed a hope that they could "shake down" what they had learned thus far and allow space for our presentation to be helpful. Our met-aphor may have been effective, as several participants later commented that the presentation allowed them to "bring it all together" into a unified whole. The creation of a solid therapeutic foundation in both psychotherapy and hypnosis should probably happen in much the same way. It involves the attainment and assimilation of new skills through continued education, supervised practice, and an openness and willingness to learn from both professionals and clients.

Expertise
One critical way to assure that hypnotherapy will remain both an ethical and valuable extension of your skills is to practice only within your areas and level of expertise. As we will often remind you, hyp-nosis should be used only to treat those conditions that a therapist would be prepared to treat without hypnosis. This is one critical way by which you will preserve your uninhibited integration of hypnosis and preserve the quality of your work. If you typically work with children, it would follow that this is a population with which you would use hypnosis. Likewise, if you are experienced working with clinical depression and anxiety, these too would be symptom constellations for which you could consider hypnotic interventions. If a therapist wishes to use hypnosis to treat a disorder with which he is not familiar, he should first become competent treating that condition before attempt-ing to utilize hypnosis.

Continued Education
This brings us to the subject of continuing education. We would guess that, if everyone who took a beginning hypnosis workshop regularly attended advanced trainings, they would be overflowing with partic-ipants. They are not. We suspect that psychotherapists new to hypnosis are sometimes unaware of the extent to which continued education

will substantially add to their competence. They might believe that, by seeking supervision or continued training, they are acknowledging a weakness in their skills. Well, we would have to agree. It is when we decide we know everything that we soon discover how little we do know. Imagine the ballet dancer learning a dramatically new step and discontinuing her classes before understanding how this step will fit into her style or be important to broader pieces of choreography. With hypnosis, we continue to learn simply because there are so many variations, styles, and applications. We have found that our illustrious Individualized Consultation faculty at ASCH's Annual Meetings routinely strive to attend as many of the other presentations as possible. In conducting our seminars and certification workshops for ASCH, we have been delighted with the opportunity to learn from the breadth of knowledge and experience of our diverse participants. A true master is first and always a student.

Healthy Boundaries
Again, what we are expecting of the clinician is good, common clinical sense. Our codes of ethical conduct concerning patient care emphasize that the well-being of the individual client be held in highest regard, by using "meaningful, professional contact with each patient" (Hammond & Elkins, 1994). We maintain that we have never really seen any harm come from the inclusion of hypnosis in treatment when conducted by a responsible therapist. "Responsible" is the critical word here. Unfortunately, we hear of situations where unscrupulous therapists have used their clinical skills to exert an unhealthy advantage over their clients. Hypnotic techniques, in the hands of such individuals, can be of particular harm to vulnerable and trusting clients.

The foundation of both ethical and effective hypnosis lies in the therapist consistently and diligently working to use hypnosis in an ethical, clear-cut way. Not only are our clients *always* well educated and prepared for hypnosis, but taking these steps also facilitates a sound therapeutic rapport that makes the work safe and comfortable for them. We must always consider the client's mental status, boundaries, sensitivities, belief systems, and wishes before beginning safe, ethical, and effective treatment.

Another boundary concern in hypnotherapy is the complex issue of touching. It is an acceptable practice for physicians and dentists to routinely touch their patients. Consequently, hypnotic methods that require limited physical contact are not met with surprise or excessive discomfort. Psychotherapists, on the other hand, must be very careful about having physical contact with their clients. As a matter of general practice, we restrict touching our clients to only handshakes or maybe a pat on the back with children in the presence of their parents. We otherwise allow our golden retrievers, Shamus and Sweetie, to provide the tactile nurturing that some clients might need.

The wish to use certain hypnotic techniques forces us to challenge these limits. Some therapists, who would never otherwise touch a client, might wish to use arm levitation or glove anesthesia for the purpose of demonstrating hypnotic phenomena or deepening trance. Yet unexpected emotional revelations and repressed conflicts with intimacy may preclude a client's readiness for touch.

We advise informing our clients of our wish to include touch and always *asking for permission* to do so. Even then, we must consider that a willingness to be touched could reflect a desire to be accommodating and not truly represent a client's underlying emotional state. Therefore, hypnosis involving touch is best utilized after *proper rapport* is established. If a client presents with discomfort about hypnosis, therapy, or even self-discovery, these boundaries must be observed until safety and stability are sufficiently restored. The first goal of trauma work is to stabilize the person's ego functioning and resilience to both external and internal stressors (Brown & Fromm, 1986).

Expectations
One additional means of assuring an ethical and relaxed approach to hypnosis is to simply maintain reasonable expectations. It is not unusual for a therapist practicing hypnosis to have clients who request and expect the "quick cure." By accepting such an impossible assignment, he would guarantee failure for himself and his client. I (RV) recently received a call from a man suffering from agoraphobia but who was, admittedly, uncomfortable with psychotherapy. He indicated he would be willing to come for one session "if that will take care of it." It would be easy to say, "Sure, let's try." Yet, to be ethical and responsible, it was more helpful to educate this man about his misconceptions than it would have been to give him one more experience with failure. He was offered more realistic expectations for treatment and given the option of beginning his work whenever he felt ready.

The therapeutic relationship begins with the first contact. From that point, we communicate our trustworthiness and professionalism. The ease with which hypnotherapy proceeds for both parties will be influenced by this initial interaction. There is nothing to be gained by targeting outcomes or accepting responsibility for change that lies beyond the limits of a therapist's skills or a client's capacities. In using hypnosis, we wish to evoke the powers of the unconscious and initiate a new precedent for success. These outcomes alone will prove beneficial for our clients as they negotiate with themselves their readiness for change. The empowerment lies in the process; therefore the process becomes the outcome.

Special Considerations: Informed Consent and Memory

The use of informed consent is relatively new in the field of psychotherapy in general and specifically when hypnosis is included in treatment. Some therapists argue that a separate informed consent for hypnosis is unnecessary, citing that they do not have written contracts with clients specifying that they can use empathy, cognitive-behavioral treatment, or psychodynamic interpretations as part of treatment. Why, then, if hypnosis is similarly only a therapeutic tool and not a treatment per se, do we require a written agreement with a client (Hammond et al., 1995).

As we emphasized in the previous section, our clients have a need as well as a right to understand the methods that will be utilized in their treatment plan. With all of our clients, we make it a habit of explaining pretty much everything we do. In particular, hypnosis has a more colorful history than many other therapeutic tools and, thus, its mystique should be addressed fully to gain the client's trust.

Equally important are the possible legal ramifications of using hypnosis that do not exist with other interventions. Due to controversy regarding the accuracy of memories elicited through hypnosis, most states have statutes restricting the testimony in court by individuals who have been hypnotized (Hammond et al., 1995). Thus, if the therapist suspects a trauma history, the client's legal rights might best be protected by not using hypnosis. At the very least, informed consent involves sharing this dilemma with your client and allowing him to make his own decision.

The reader might wonder how the addition of a thorough informed consent will help to make using hypnosis more comfortable. We find that the novice hypnotherapist often fears making clinical or ethical mistakes that will result in failure or legal consequences. Although these fears are largely unnecessary, or at least exaggerated, they will inhibit the free and creative application of hypnosis. For this reason, we believe that the reporting of informed consent issues at the outset of hypnotherapy is helpful in dispelling the myths that elicit apprehensions for both therapist and client. This presentation needs to be comprehensive yet reassuring in order to ease anxieties and not nurture them.

Hypnosis offers the potential to access previously repressed emotions and memories more easily than with most types of psychotherapy (Hammond et al., 1995). We introduce hypnosis to treatment with the hope that additional, consciously unavailable information might be accessed. The focus of our treatment then becomes a function not only of fact but also perhaps of perception, interpretation, and distortion.

It is not uncommon for a clinician to wonder whether a client who presents with dissociative symptoms might have a history of trauma. While a thorough diagnostic interview should include such queries, we know that traumatic memories could possibly be repressed, only to surface later. A client could initially present with a simple phobia, headaches, or performance anxiety, and then, in later therapy sessions, we discover that a trauma history lurks at the root of these symptoms. At that point it would be too late for her to make an informed decision. For that reason, we advise that all clients be given full and accurate information about hypnosis and the possible ramifications of its use.

However, because hypnosis has been singled out as having potential legal ramifications for the client, we make it a routine practice to discuss these possible consequences with our clients. A client seeking hypnotherapy for smoking cessation or performance anxiety might appear to be unlikely to uncover traumatic memories, so you might be tempted to omit "advised consent" from your procedures. Clients should always be made aware of this prior to beginning hypnosis, regardless of whether such histories are suspected — you never know.

Therefore, all hypnosis clients should be educated about the nature of memory and how it is possibly influenced by various environmental, interpersonal, and intrapersonal factors. Whether memories arise spontaneously or as the result of a therapeutic intervention, we cannot assume that they are unbiased recollections of past events. We also know that memories can be altered by leading questions in or out of hypnosis (Hammond et al., 1995). While stressing that you do not doubt their perceptions of events or reports of emotional injury, you must make it clear that any memories that might be recovered will likely be clouded and distorted at best. The legal implications of this inexactness need to be emphasized as well. Any therapeutic intervention must take into account the individual needs, fears, and expectations of the client.

A good resource for dealing with this issue is the handbook *Clinical Hypnosis and Memory: Guidelines for Clinicians and for Forensic Hypnosis* (Hammond et al., 1995), by the ASCH Committee on Hypnosis and Memory. In addition, being informed about the ethics codes provided by your state and professional organizations will help you to feel confident and comfortable with your decision-making.

CHAPTER 2

The Hypnotic Relationship

THE FUNDAMENTALS

In December of 2000, I (RV) moved from Massachusetts to Brunswick, Maine, and began to transition my long-standing practice to a new hometown. Given the size of my caseload and the lengthy tenure of several clients, I understood that a few terminations could and should take months to complete. After my move, I drove to Massachusetts weekly to see these clients until they had all completed their work or termination. Carla had been my client off and on for years. She has most recently been treated for early childhood trauma and a dissociative disorder that had not at first been evident. Hypnosis was a regular part of her treatment as we visited and learned from the various, estranged corners of her unconscious.

Given the severity of her condition, I broached with her the possibility of a transfer to another local psychotherapist once my trips to Massachusetts had ended. To say that she was distressed and angry would be an understatement. As I expressed my concern and pressed the point of a transfer, she slapped her knee and with tearful exasperation said, "Do you know how long it takes to train a therapist?" Carla decided to make the two-hour drive and continue to see me in my Brunswick office.

Well, so much for sound clinical judgment. While I thought I was being conscientious and looking out for Carla's better interests, I overlooked what was obviously the most important ingredient to her improvement (obvious to her, anyway). She reminded me that the relationship we had built over our years together could not be easily recreated with someone else and that she would not easily surrender her trust in me to geographical inconvenience. It is perhaps this chemistry, not my skills, that has contributed most to her significant improvement.

Utilizing hypnosis to communicate with one's unconscious makes treatment an intimate and extraordinary experience. Psychological boundaries become more fluid and diffuse. Metaphorically, your client is not only inviting you into her house, but is allowing you the liberty of accessing the closets, basement, and attic as well. I (RV) had spent considerable time inside Carla's "house" and proven myself worthy of the invitation. She was not about to allow someone else the freedom she had bestowed upon me. This is an honor we must respect and protect at all times.

We reiterate here that the effectiveness of any psychotherapy lies in the integrity of the relationship in which it occurs. That integrity consists of sound clinical training, consistently good ethics and judgment, residence within one's strengths and expertise, and the development of dynamic and fluid therapeutic communication. Hypnosis will fit much more easily into treatment when you remain within these parameters. There is simply less perceived risk for both therapist and client when hypnosis is introduced into such a strong foundation. As we review the following fundamental elements to a healthy therapeutic relationship, we hope you will recognize their contributions in facilitating the integration of hypnosis into practice.

Trust

A physician friend (MD) believes that the greatest need people have is to be understood. In the process of psychotherapy, one of the most beneficial and comforting aspects throughout treatment is that of being accurately heard and unconditionally accepted. These qualities also characterize the trust and rapport that is the foundation of all psychotherapeutic work. Given popular misconceptions about hypnosis and the intimate nature of the hypnotic session, the creation of sound trust and rapport becomes an even more important stage of treatment. Regardless of the viability of the therapeutic relationship when hypnosis begins, its introduction will likely challenge a client's trust in her therapist and treatment itself. By agreeing to use hypnosis, it is as though your client is saying she will accept help not only on a level she understands (conscious), but also on a level she does not (unconscious).

Furthermore, in all relationships, trust must be earned. It is critical that the hypnotherapist evaluate what his client might need to cultivate her trust and to engage her in whatever course of action this involves. After my initial work with Susan (RV) had seemingly established a solid basis of a common language and clear goals, I suggested to her that we begin using hypnosis to help her manage emerging sadness and rage from an early childhood experience. She arrived at our next session and asked, "Will you humor me?" "Sure," I said. She proceeded to line up various rocks and crystals on my coffee table and then lit a dried sage bundle that filled my office with a wonderful scent. Upon completing her ritual, she simply stated, "Okay, now we can begin." When asked her reasons for all this, she just added, "It will help me trust you."

While many dependent or desperate clients might rush into a therapeutic relationship, trusting too quickly and exposing themselves to unfortunate and unnecessary risk and harm, we must maintain and model a respect for their and our own safety and personal integrity through our establishing and observing appropriate healthy boundaries. We must be required to earn their trust and deserve this gift once it is given.

From a more practical standpoint, a trusting client is a less resistant one. While the allure of power might draw a therapist to learn hypnosis, it is the demystification of this power that produces a more willing and invested subject. A patient and thorough investment in gaining their trust fortified my relationships with Carla and Susan. As a result, our work flowed freely as I reached often to apply the soft brush of hypnosis.

Rapport

All hypnotherapy is, by nature, client-centered. A therapist must recognize and honor the person before him unconditionally by respecting enduring symptoms as important and integral facets of survival and adaptation, however unhealthy they might seem. Therefore, hypnosis must begin by properly understanding the client and deciding on a course of treatment that is manageable and takes into account all conscious and unconscious motivations. From this stance emerge empathy and rapport.

Through the manifestation of your interpersonal style, experiential training, and clinical experience, you readily create empathic connections with your clients. Although the process is ostensibly the same, the establishment of rapport in hypnosis carries broader implications. In a way, rapport provides the basis for the hypnotherapeutic relationship. As we reflect our clients' behavior and words, we form an unconscious bond that will later become the foundation for hypnotic intervention. The language of rapport matures into the language of induction.

Two key strategies in communicating empathy and building rapport are *mirroring* and *accurate feedback*. These are simple means by which you can effortlessly join with your client in the creation of a common language and shared experience. As you begin using hypnosis, you will do so from a position that is reflective of their current state and, thus, familiar and congruent for them. In fact, these techniques can make the introduction of hypnosis much smoother and easier to accomplish.

Mirroring (Gilligan, 1987; Grinder & Bandler, 1981) is a common component of everyday human interaction. One only needs to go sit in a restaurant and observe couples dining together. Those who unconsciously mimic each other's behaviors will most likely have the deepest rapport. You will notice how their gestures, head nods, eye movements, and even changes in facial tone reflect one another. A comical example of mirroring is found in the movie *Twins* (1988). Danny DeVito and Arnold Schwarzenegger portray an unusual set of fraternal twins. Upon their reunion, they discover their commonalities in a lovely depiction of mirrored behavior. Despite their obviously contrasting physical attributes, the two men sit at dinner with identical ways of seasoning and savoring their meals.

Beginning therapists are taught how to mirror their clients with posture, gesture, and facial expression. As we gain experience, this practice becomes a spontaneous result of our attention and observation. For example, during a marital therapy session I (RV) was conducting with another therapist, I noticed that the wife's hands were clasped in a rather unusual way, thumbs joined and moving from an internal rhythm. As I scanned down, I noticed that not only were my co-therapist's hands and thumbs in the same position, but mine were also.

What is important to understand is that mirroring not only facilitates rapport, but is also a critical facet of hypnotic language. From a naturalistic standpoint, your conscious and unconscious efforts to reflect your client's behavior through your words and actions establish the foundation for hypnotic induction and intervention. It is as though your client engages you with a subtle invitation to dance and you just as subtly accept.

Accurate Feedback

If mirroring is our method of reflecting our clients' physical behavior, the giving of accurate feedback is meant to echo their words and their stories. As we discovered in our graduate training, empathy can be learned. Whereas compassion might be more a product of our upbringing and life experiences, listening involves skill and attentiveness. Perhaps "hearing" is a melding of both. We recall from our early education those exercises when we were asked to reflect what our role-playing clients said to us. Gradually, our comments took on greater depth and accuracy. Our case supervision involved honing these skills while we also developed greater insight into our countertransference and roots of understanding.

As we regularly practice these skills, we become more aware of nuances in our clients' communication and learn to respond with greater precision and depth of understanding. By combining accurate physical and verbal feedback, we build the rapport to support less-intrusive hypnotic interaction. We begin to fashion suggestions that feel congruent for our clients. In speaking and mirroring truths of a client's present experience, we are validating that experience while also eliciting his internal frame of reference. For example, matching a client's breathing is one of the simplest and most fundamental ways to initiate rapport and hypnotic communication (Gilligan, 1987). You are literally in sync with a most basic physiological function. What better way to walk in another's shoes than to share their breath?

Amanda, a young mother of twins, was referred by her physician for anxiety. She spoke in a breathless, hurried manner as she described the chaos of her life. She complained that even prior to the appearance of her babies, she had felt overwhelmed by the details of life. As I (MD) matched her breathing pattern, I became increasingly aware of the scattered way in which she described her situation. A sense of confusion, not anxiety, began to envelop me. If anything, anxiety was secondary to the sense of being in the midst of a mental cyclone. Further questioning of Amanda's history revealed that she had many of the hallmarks of adult attention deficit disorder. Matching her breathing had put us in sync with one another, allowing an accurate diagnosis to emerge. Because of her difficulties with attention, fractionation was a wonderful hypnotic intervention. Fractionation matched

Amanda's innate ability to focus toward and away from stimuli and was thus very useful in helping her enter very deep and productive states of trance.

Our intention here is not to rehash basic communication skills. Rather, we want our readers to view such skills as a stage in the hypnotic process. In hypnotic terms, mirroring and accurate feedback become the basis for naturalistic language and trance induction. Perhaps more importantly, the genuineness you project through such attention to detail brings your client closer to you. She will become more likely to trust you and herself in learning new and more difficult steps together.

Building Cooperation and Hope

One strategy that will both reflect the true nature of hypnosis and prevent unnecessary fears of failure is to view everything the client does as successful. In Erickson's early work, he observed that clients would sometimes produce "coincidental [hypnotic] phenomena" (Rossi, 1993) in addition to those that he had suggested. His simple conclusion was that the unconscious has the capacity to manifest expressions unique to the individual and that this information could be useful in treatment. While we might seek a certain, curative outcome to hypnosis, we need not be invested in our client's idiosyncratic responses as we work toward those ends. Rather, client behavior during hypnosis should be considered revealing and informative, not a measure of success or failure. Moreover, should the therapist anticipate which client response is correct, she would also be assuming responsibility for trance and hypnotic behavior. We know that this would be a false assumption, rife with the potential for anxiety and failure. The mission is to provide opportunities for the client's unconscious to participate in treatment, not to direct what that participation will be.

Behind this view of hypnotic behavior and therapist expectation lies the supposition that a person's unconscious mind controls his body, behavior, thinking, and mood. Therefore, we can assume that virtually all qualities of a client's presentation or functioning originate in the unconscious (Rossi & Cheek, 1988). We can further assume that, because the unconscious strives for healing and survival, its manifestations during hypnosis will be implicitly constructive (Rossi, 1993). By using hypnosis, we access those layers of our client's thinking and behavior that go beyond their usual linear (conscious) ways of thinking and functioning to something more fundamentally helpful to understanding and growth. The challenge lies in utilizing these expressions therapeutically. As you adapt the attitude of "creative indifference" with your clients, the function and therapeutic potentials of these expressions become more understandable and adaptable.

It has been our experience that nothing inhibits the neophyte hypnotherapist more than the fear of saying the "wrong" thing. Anxiety about using the "correct" language or creating the "perfect" metaphor shifts the focus onto the therapist and inhibits him from adapting his own words, ideas, and style. A clumsy and rigid adherence to words that overemphasize relaxation and little else prevent the hypnotherapist from speaking in a genuine and responsive manner. Effective hypnosis is "self-less" on the part of the therapist. That is, the less you try to be perfect or clever and instead attend to what your client gives you, the more successful your work will be.

In the course of our work, we are often surprised by which of our comments clients discover to have the most impact. Perhaps we have made an offhanded comment that the client has interpreted or incorporated in some meaningful way. It is impossible to predict which words or interactions our clients will find to be the most significant, regardless of the mode of psychotherapy we are using. Not only do we rarely worry about this happening, we usually learn something of value about our clients in the process. Why then, when using a tool such as hypnosis, should we feel such a need to control our words and the impressions they leave?

At the conclusion of a recent beginning hypnosis workshop that had featured several different instructors, we were delighted to hear a psychotherapist from the South exclaim, "Wow, everybody does this differently. Y'all just are yourselves when you do hypnosis." For the most part, she was correct. Although we all seek to induce and exploit the benefits of trance, our points of intervention, choice of words, and interpersonal styles will always be unique. Overemphasis on language and a belief that hypnosis needs to be practiced in a particular way can cause even seasoned hypnotherapists to ignore the very opportunities that can make hypnosis a relatively natural process.

PREPARING YOUR CLIENT:
MYTHS AND MISCONCEPTIONS

Clients who are new to hypnosis often carry with them many misconceptions and apprehensions about what will happen *to* them. Their success in enjoying and benefiting from hypnosis will likely be greatly influenced by their expectations and readiness to trust in the therapist's lead. Therefore, hypnosis should begin with a straightforward review of exactly what is about to transpire. What is trance? How will it help? If trance is a focused, absorbed state of consciousness, how does hypnosis work in achieving it?

In order to answer these and other questions, I (RV) have prepared an article on the myths and misconceptions about hypnosis. We both often refer clients to our Web site (delaneyandvoit.com), where they can read this article and a great deal more about hypnosis and the training of hypnotherapists. Prior to beginning hypnosis, we take great care in reviewing not only what trance is, but also what it isn't. Examples of natural trance are given, reinforcing an understanding that what they are about to experience will be somehow natural and familiar. The induction of choice is described in advance and its rationale is explained. The power and effectiveness of hypnosis is not improved with mystery and surprise, but by confidence and safety.

We routinely ask our clients what their present view of hypnosis is and how they viewed hypnosis as children. Most clients have had some exposure to hypnosis in the media. If this began in their childhood, part of their belief system may still carry a perception gleaned from some comedic or melodramatic portrayal. In either case, it is helpful to know what kinds of early, distorted ideas they may have about hypnosis.

We are also particularly interested in knowing whether they have attended a stage hypnosis performance, which might have created grossly inaccurate misconceptions about the potential for embarrassment or a sudden, unwelcome loss of control. If the client has seen such a presentation, we emphasize that, in a stage performance, the hypnotist is primarily interested in providing entertainment and that the participants are expecting to be embarrassed. We further reassure them that the stage hypnotist routinely asks the audience to perform certain tasks to determine which individuals might be the most suggestible. He then asks for volunteers and only selects those who appear to be very good subjects. It has been rumored that the hypnotist also has confederates in the audience who become "volunteers" for the demonstration. We advise that stage hypnosis differs greatly from what we do as therapists. Our intention is not to control or embarrass our clients, but rather to act as their partner and guide them toward growth and relief.

Misconceptions about hypnosis are also the basis for doubts regarding its usefulness. Most newly trained hypnotherapists likely dread the prospect of hearing a client assert, "I don't think I can be hypnotized!" Such a declaration might leave the therapist fearing that resistance will limit his client's responsiveness to hypnosis. However, such apprehensions should neither be received as a personal challenge to the therapist nor as a permanent barrier to successful hypnosis. It is more likely that these statements represent a client's anxiety about her own performance or concerns for her psychological safety. These reservations simply teach us that this person needs more preparation and that hypnotic language should be geared toward managing resistance. As therapists, we need to welcome our clients' concerns and questions regarding hypnosis and to address them as we would any other treatment issue.

As a general practice, to reduce client anxiety and resistance, we have found it most helpful to identify and underscore the following tenets regarding hypnosis:

Trance is a naturally occurring state of consciousness that we will access through hypnotic techniques. In many ways, trance is like a daydream. Everyone has had the experience of "drifting off" during a boring lecture or while driving a car. In hypnosis, we purposely induce the same "ability" to absorb and focus our attention. This allows their unconscious, creative, problem-solving potentials to become more available. When first introducing hypnotic induction, I (RV) usually attempt to elicit a pleasant, uncomplicated trance with suggestions that will connect my client to other times they may have felt the same experience. I emphasize how they will not only remember those times of such a peaceful calm, but that they will also learn to recognize them in the future. This practice in itself usually eliminates my clients' doubts and fears while handing them full control and a requisite responsibility for the trance itself.

The client is always in control during the hypnosis. Clients need to know that they are in control of what happens in their treatment as a whole and particularly with hypnosis. It can be reassuring for them to know that they can not only regulate the depth and breadth of their experience, but that in many respects they actually have more control during hypnosis. In my (RV) early hypnotic work with one dissociative client, she related that she was frightened by the misperception that my voice had become louder and that I had possibly moved closer to her. I simply invited her to open her eyes and leave them open as long as she wished. When asked if she felt reassured of her safety, she said,

"Yes," and closed her eyes once again. This same client later complained that one of her younger ego states did not like the classical music in my waiting room. Making use of her strong sense of humor, I suggested toward the end of a hypnotic session that she would "find a curious but enjoyable appreciation for classical music." With her eyes still closed, she simply stated, "A_ _h_ _ _!" I was able to demonstrate through this use of levity exactly how much control she had and that no part of her was lost in the process!

Clients also fear that they will also become totally oblivious to their surroundings. This is of particular concern to them as they begin to practice self-hypnosis. We remind them of other experiences in which they were deeply absorbed but able to hear naturally occurring noises such as a phone ringing or a baby crying. For example, many people have had the experience of hearing their radio alarm clock begin while remaining in a very relaxed half-sleep. They hear the news or music being broadcast and, if need be, could recall what they heard, but are nonetheless deeply absorbed in their restful state. The choice of whether or not to respond to stimuli in their environment is theirs.

The client will have control over the content — affect, memory, or behavior during the hypnotic experience. In short, it is important to reassure the client that, if they become uncomfortable with anything that occurs during hypnosis, they can: (a) reject the suggestion; (b) use finger or hand signals to indicate so; (c) speak to the therapist during hypnosis; or (d), if they prefer, bring themselves out of trance. With particularly apprehensive clients, we will often demonstrate all of these contingencies before initiating more substantial work.

To alleviate clients' anxiety (and perhaps my own), I (RV) will often demonstrate what I *do* and to not expect anything profound to occur. I ask them to close their eyes for a few minutes while I talk to them, suggest an absorption in some internal image, and allow them to open their eyes as they wish. Once again, by seeding continual reassurances of control and choice throughout hypnosis, you protect against resistance, reduce client anxiety, and ratify trance phenomena in the process. What serves the client also serves the hypnotherapist.

THERAPIST'S USE OF SELF

During one of our hypnosis seminars, it was my turn to provide a demonstration with one of the participants. I (MD) asked Christina if there was something specific she wanted to work on, with the caveat that she could keep the content of the problem private so long as we could discuss its theme. Christina asked that we work on her fertility difficulties, with a specific wish that she would carry a healthy baby to full term. Being an intimate group, several of us were already aware that she had experienced a number of miscarriages. So her request did not come as a total surprise.

Having experienced my own frustrations with this issue, my empathy for her was immediate. I'm not sure it was noticeable to Christina, but I momentarily panicked, wondering whether I could remain objective and helpful. However, I quickly realized that this was a fortuitous, if not challenging, opportunity. Christina, despite all of her painful and discouraging failures, maintained hope. Who better to help her than someone who knew this kind of disappointment from both sides? I had experienced the frustration of endless unsuccessful treatments as well as the eventual joyful appearance of a beautiful child.

Still, I had no clue what I was going to say. I bought myself some time by demonstrating embedded commands, presuppositions, and focused questions to both pace her frustrations and encourage ego strengthening. My intervention, to that point, still remained a mystery. Fortunately, my unconscious must have been listening, as the theme of frustration and rebirth brought to mind the film *Little Women* (1994), one of my (MD) all-time favorite books and movies. Specifically, I recalled the passage in which an angry Amy burns Jo's manuscript. What I love about this sequence in the story is that Jo is both absolutely livid and crushed. Like a woman whose attempts at pregnancy end in loss and failure, Jo must face the fact that her hard work and good intentions did not result in the birth of her first novel. Women struggling with infertility know this pain. They do all the "right" things with no guarantee of success. Likewise, the disappointment and anger that can accompany these failed efforts often feel toxic. Women often suppress these negative feelings in fear that they will jeopardize the very thing they are trying to do. Indeed, it is not uncommon for them to become depressed when they are unable to constructively manage their negative reactions. Like Jo upon the destruction of her manuscript, they often feel hopeless and helpless, wondering if they can muster the strength and resourcefulness to replicate their efforts once again.

I related how, while trying to accommodate her mother's request to forgive Amy, Jo's chilly veneer could not disguise her temporary hatred. It takes Amy's near-death experience, partly due to Jo's neglect,

to provide a place where the two headstrong young women can rec-
oncile. Amy promises to assist Jo in rewriting her novel, and indeed
they do, creating a work that is superior to the original.

As the tears streamed down Christina's smiling face, I had difficulty suppressing my own. Her face spoke first what post-hypnotically
she confirmed in words: that the metaphor felt "right." I silently
thanked her for her inspiration and my unconscious resources for
sharing their wisdom.

I often use this story as a metaphor in characterizing the nature
of "originality" and resourcefulness in developing an effective and
comfortable approach to hypnosis. Sometimes we don't know how
much we know until we have to use it. In other words, rather than
concentrating on doing hypnosis "the right way," begin to believe that
your skills as a therapist and your experiences in and out of work will
guide you at the times you need them most. This is not to say that
there are not specific hypnosis skills that you will want to master, but
that your concerns about technique should not overshadow a trust in
your clinical instincts and unconscious resources.

It is common that, when we adopt a new skill, we attempt to mimic
the words and style of our teachers. In our teaching we have found
this to be especially true when therapists are first learning hypnosis.
For years I (MD) worried that I would never have the command of
language and metaphor that Erickson, Gilligan, and my other teachers
seemed to possess. The unfortunate consequence of such an attitude
was that it prevented me from utilizing my most important resources —
my clients and myself. My development as a hypnotherapist began
when I assigned responsibility for trance behavior to my clients and
when I assumed responsibility for my own language, metaphor, and
style. It is from the blending and weaving of these two rich reserves
that the dynamics of hypnosis evolve.

In this way, the process of therapy is often like dancing. Two people
connect and begin to move to their own shared melody. This is just a
fanciful way of saying that when a therapist and her client engage, there
is a potential for much more to occur than "what meets the ears." The
client brings all her spoken and unspoken beliefs, hopes, and fears, while
the therapist contributes his skill, warmth, and understanding. Over
the course of treatment, through a myriad of words, postures, facial
expressions, and even silence, two new partners begin the dance,
fusing styles and timing their steps to their own distinctive melody.

Over the past six years, the authors have discussed many of our
own cases with each other and have taught numerous seminars

together. In the process, we have become quite familiar with each other's work and have discovered that we share a common psychotherapeutic orientation and view of the hypnotic process. This book is a reflection of the extent to which our philosophies and professional interests mesh. At the same time, we have recognized that our styles of actually practicing hypnosis differ considerably. Those differences are rooted in our disparate personal histories, tastes, associations, and interpersonal styles. Knowing each other as well as we do, our hypnotic language and pacing have gradually become more similar. Concurrently, we are also able to recognize how each other's clinical idiosyncrasies reveal more about personal characteristics than psychological orientation.

The practice of psychotherapy is one of the most creative professions in the healing arts. It is a unique combination of skill, knowledge, and the use of self as instruments for growth. The addition of hypnosis to your repertoire can greatly enhance the potential of creative thinking and expression in your therapeutic work. The dancer who perfects his steps and routines ultimately moves to his own internal rhythm. We encourage our readers to know and use themselves the same way in the practice of hypnosis.

CHAPTER 3

Beginning Treatment: What Our Clients Teach Us about Themselves

Each clinician develops his own procedure and style in diagnosing a new client. This can include everything from a formal psychometric assessment to reliance upon "gut" instincts. We often refer to *DSM-IV* (1994) guidelines for diagnosis, particularly when it is necessary to write a report or submit insurance claims. Our diagnoses usually are inclusive of a client's presenting complaints but must also be comprehensive of her overall mental status.

An accurate assessment is critical, because it will answer several important questions. First, and perhaps most importantly, is this a client that fits within my areas of expertise? Secondly, at what level of readiness for change does this client enter treatment? This will determine the nature of our initial client education and intervention. Finally, what clinical tools do I practice that will be most helpful in relieving symptoms and, hopefully, resolving the diagnosis? As we reviewed earlier, our courses of action will also be directed by our clinical orientation and even personal philosophies.

Obviously, our initial impressions can change as we learn more about an individual and as she gains sufficient trust to disclose the more guarded facets of her story. Our treatment plan should never be so narrow and inflexible as to prevent a smooth adjustment to new information. The more confidence we have in our diagnostic impressions and in our own skills, the more effective treatment will be.

We have previously stressed the point that, when we have a clear clinical picture of our clients and remain within our breadth of expertise, the introduction of hypnosis becomes much more comfortable and successful. At this point, we would like to outline a means of diagnosing a client in ways that will further enhance this comfort and success. The key to integrating hypnosis into practice is through the translation of our clients' characteristics and hypnotic phenomena into effective treatment strategies.

Everything our clients do, think, feel, and imagine offers us valuable inroads into their unconscious processes. We are routinely reading and responding to our clients' facial expressions, body language, and other idiosyncratic behaviors. The movies they watch, the music they prefer, and the way they dress all reflect an internal world that is long-standing and durable. These "messages" from the unconscious offer valuable information about internal conflicts, mood, and readiness for suggestion.

Therefore, our usual diagnostic methods are inadequate to identify or categorize such information, which is as idiosyncratic as our clients themselves. When we must begin to look at our clients through "fresh eyes" the pathways to hypnotic intervention will appear.

Here we will suggest areas of our clients' presentation that might be useful in beginning hypnotic assessment.

GENERAL CHARACTERISTICS: WINDOWS
TO THE UNCONSCIOUS

Psychotherapists are trained observers. We spend the better part of an hour with focused attention on every nuance of our clients' words and behavior. On conscious and unconscious levels, whether we know it or not, we hear their stories and absorb the subtleties of their presence. If we should attend only to their complaints and concern ourselves with explicit diagnostic impressions, we will miss much of the valuable information they provide.

The following is a list of potential attributes of hypnotic value. It is by no means complete, as the possibilities are virtually endless.

General Characteristics

1. **Attire** — preferred colors, attention to detail, formal/casual, tight/loose
2. **Avocations** — sports, exercise, crafts, reading
3. **Interests** — musical tastes, animals, travel, writing
4. **Employment** — indoor/outdoor, technical, artistic, medical
5. **Tastes** — music, food, art, movies
6. **Physical traits** — athletic, over/underweight, hairstyle, demonstrative

Carla is an accountant for a telemarketing firm. She has worked with numbers for most of her adult life and there is little doubt she is very good at what she does. But that is not Carla. She is a person who loves nature. Much of her free time is spent walking the trails of local forests and state parks. She feeds the birds and watches quietly when a family of deer strolls through a clearing. Her dreams are of rivers, woods, and sensations of the day's weather. She brings biscuits to my (RV) dog and strokes his hair as she talks. Carla has numerous medical problems that create fairly constant physical discomfort and occasional acute pain. She believes that it is her will that allows her to function and to ultimately heal. Her history is filled with physical and emotional trauma and she suffers from a dissociative identity disorder.

What does this tell us about Carla and the potential for hypnotic intervention? First of all, we know that a trauma history and dissociative disorders are highly correlated with hypnotizability. Yet because of her trauma history, we would pay close attention to boundaries and creating a perception of safety. Therefore, her induction should be permissive, naturalistic, and relatively simple, with an initial focus upon ego strengthening and suggestions for safety. She will be responsive to direct suggestion, but must always be given choices and control. We know that she will be receptive to suggestions emphasizing visual beauty and texture. She will be more drawn to images from the outdoors, wildlife, and climate. Her awareness of physical sensation will be keen, while some areas of emotional insight could be limited. We might borrow a few terms from accounting such as "balance" or "making things add up."

We find that the longer we practice psychotherapy, the more automatically we mirror and reflect our clients' presentation. They slouch, we slouch. They speak softly, we speak softly. Even these general characteristics creep into our language without conscious awareness. With the addition of hypnosis, we merely suggest that you can pay even closer attention to useful detail.

ASSESSING AND UTILIZING SENSORY STRENGTHS

Each of us has a preferred method of embracing the world and incorporating the information we receive through our worldview (Gilligan, 1987). Some of us are primarily *visual* in our orientation: we *see* the big picture or we can *focus* on the details of a situation. Others of us rely most heavily on our *auditory* sensory system such that we *hear* what someone is telling us or we can *listen* easily to the ideas of others or to the *voice* in our mind. Some of us are more tied into our *kinesthetic* system so that we are more *sensitive* to the feelings of others, or we can *feel comfortable* with a new experience (Gilligan, 1987; Grinder, Delozier & Bandler, 1977; Mills & Crowley, 1986).

We use all three of these sensory systems to some degree. Typically, we are strongest in one modality, followed by a second preferred system. Musicians, for example, are often primarily auditory, followed by either kinesthetic or visual. Someone who is primarily visual may hear classical music and imagine a beautiful ballet. The music is secondary to the scenes she is creating in her mind. The primarily kinesthetic person may find it difficult to be in crowded places, as they are more sensitized to how a space "feels."

The identification of a client's primary sensory systems will enhance hypnotic communication and the choice of imagery (Gilligan, 1987; Mills & Crowley, 1986). Matching your language to your client's representational system will contribute greatly to establishing rapport and hypnotic communication. However, accurately hearing and tailoring your suggestions to a client's sensory style can sometimes be challenging. For example, George (from Chapter 1) was very hypnotizable, suggestible, and comfortable with hypnosis but was having trouble with the visual imagery I (RV) had initially used. When left to his own imagination, he was unable to see much of anything during hypnosis. The color, movement, and pathways I was providing were simply difficult to see. Recalling that George was a college teacher and textbook author, I decided to suggest that he see a book and that the pages would open to one in particular that would provide the *words* of some significance to his problem. In reading the words, he was able to *hear* the message he needed to hear.

If it is difficult to discern your client's representational style, it is helpful to begin hypnosis with a guided imagery and suggest the use of all senses in his fantasized experience. Afterwards, by asking what parts of his imagery were most vivid, you will usually gauge his most powerful system. With other clients, we will simply suggest "closing your eyes there in your special place and sensing your surroundings...in just the right way." The details of their experience will help in identifying their preferred representational systems, and this new information can steer you in choosing corresponding hypnotic language.

Understanding our own sensory preferences is important, as it serves not only as our individual avenue of comprehending information but also as for a gateway to incorporating new knowledge. The sensory systems that we favor serve as a filter that colors both the information we receive as well as what we project out onto the environment. Being attuned to your sensory preferences will help you understand when you might be missing something in an interaction. For example, if you tend to think in visual images and your client is complaining that you aren't *hearing* them, you may be using the wrong "language" with them. They probably favor thought and ideas (auditory) as a way to understand their experience, while you are *imagining* what they are saying! Thus, understanding and identifying a client's primary sensory systems will enhance rapport, hypnotic communication, and the choice of imagery.

Being primarily visual, followed by kinesthetic, I (MD) can most easily see and feel what my clients are communicating. Often, the most challenging clients for me are those whose primary system is auditory. Without being conscious of it, I am working so diligently yet unsuccessfully to hear their message that I lose touch with my own tracking system: my pictures and feelings. Since these are what I rely upon the most, ignoring them can present barriers to accurate understanding. In other words, do not enter your client's world so completely that you lose access to your own. Conversely, use caution not to be so totally immersed in your own sensory systems that you are unable to follow those of your client.

This process is fruitful and yet not without its difficulties. While I (MD) was meeting recently with a woman for the first time, she described her medical status in very grave terms. Recent intrusive cancer surgery had been unsuccessful and inoperable cancerous tumors remained. Her condition was quite serious. Yet her words

Table 3.1
Common Sensory Language

Visual	Auditory	Kinesthetic
see	hear	hold
get the picture	listen	touch
reflect	roar	feel
viewpoint	tune in	hurt
perspective	tune out	stuck
focus	talking	electric
glow	sound	angry
color	static	falling
brighten	dialogue	sensitive
darken	conversation	grasp
colorful	loud	smooth
watch	quiet	rough
visualize	murmur	hold onto
foggy	speaking	letting go
appears	rumble	relaxed
blur	whisper	comfortable
looks like	scream	uncomfortable
photographic	sounds to me	solid
the way I look at it	listen to me	sense
see what I mean?	tone	shivers
	hear what I mean?	do you feel what I mean?

indicated that she held out hope for recovery and that she was viewing me, in part, as a way to increase her chances. As I mirrored this woman's posture and communication, suddenly a voice in my head shouted, "You are sitting with a dead person!" Since I am primarily visual and kinesthetic, I have learned that this voice typically emerges when I am missing an important communication from my client. I was listening to her words that were expressing hope, while my "voice" was translating a very dire message. I felt guilty thinking this, as if I were passing a death sentence on this client.

In consulting with Dr. Voit about my reactions, he suggested that perhaps this woman was telling me something through our empathic connection. For example, she consciously wanted very much to survive and perhaps was not at present able to face the possibility that she might die. The facts of her situation and her nonverbal (unconscious) behavior seemed to indicate that her situation was hopeless. Because my sensory strengths are visual/kinesthetic, the voice in my head mirrored those possibilities. Yet I was missing the will to live that her words expressed. Although my initial reaction may have been premature, it allowed me to "hear" an unconscious, nonverbal communication from my client. By tuning in to my intuitions rather than rejecting them, and eventually responding to her words as well, I was able to create a deeper rapport with my client as well as develop ideas for an appropriate course of treatment.

IDEOMOTOR COMMUNICATION

We wish to make a distinction here between ideomotor communication and the hypnotic technique of ideomotor signaling. By ideomotor communication we are referring to the spontaneous, nonverbal ways in which our bodies communicate emotions and/or ideas, often outside of our conscious control or even awareness. Ideomotor signaling is often used during hypnosis as a means for the therapist and client to communicate with the client's unconscious. We will provide a brief overview of this tool as a helpful response to client resistance in chapter 6. Our present focus is ideomotor communication.

The term "ideomotor" simply refers to a person's body revealing something that his words will not (Erickson et al., 1981; Yapko, 1995). Bypassing and even betraying conscious intent, physical manifestations of unconscious process defy one's defenses and speak the truth. Therapists commonly hear a client's words saying one thing, such as, "Oh, my marriage is great," while she shakes her head from side to side in contradiction.

An interesting study of ideomotor communication can be found in David Mamet's movie *House of Games* (1987), about con men. As portrayed in this film, con men describe these ideomotor behaviors as "tells." They closely observe their intended victim to assess what "tells" might give away any emotion of which they might take advantage. They learn that when a poker player unconsciously plays with his ring he is probably anxious and, therefore, bluffing.

Ideomotor communication is essentially dissociative in nature, as it represents emotions that have become detached or repressed. Whether or not we respond to these phenomena, we gain an advantage in building rapport, creating empathy, and determining a direction for treatment. We can utilize this knowledge toward trance induction and reconnecting a client with powerful but previously inaccessible information.

Kathy (RV) was a rising star in the world of high tech. She began her career as an administrative assistant but rode her intelligence and initiative to oversee product design and marketing. But a problem arose whenever she was asked to give a demonstration or lecture to a large group of her colleagues. Kathy would blush a deep red from her cheeks to the base of her neck. She didn't need a mirror, for she could feel the warmth of the blood rushing to her skin. Despite her conscious wish to perform well and advance professionally, she was revealing a contradictory message. Her embarrassment and frustration caused her to avoid and, thus, not benefit from the truth her body exposed.

Early in her life, Kathy had learned that it was safer to be unnoticed in a tense, alcoholic household. She and her brother did not want to draw the attention of her emotionally abusive father or add to the stress of her overwhelmed mother. As an adult, despite physical beauty and an engaging personality, she shunned the spotlight that she warranted. Consequently, her social life suffered as well. Kathy's unconscious expressed this aversion to attention that belied her healthy adult endeavors.

Her hypnotic protocol would begin and end with ideomotor communication. We began with an eye fixation and involuntary (dissociative) eye closure (for trance ratification). Once her eyes were fully closed, as we would expect, Kathy began to blush. The knowledge that my focus was on her evoked the same unconscious response that haunted her at work. Instead of challenging this hypnotic talent, I chose to make use of it. After asking her to attribute a number to the warmth in her face, I asked if she could increase that number by one. She indicated that she had (by finger signaling). I then asked if she could return to the original number. She did. I then asked if she would allow herself to *reduce* that number by one, two numbers. She signaled yes. A few moments later, as a smile replaced her blush, she signaled again that she had achieved a new self-control over this dreaded, archaic survival skill — a skill she no longer needed.

Ideomotor communications are simply further windows to the unconscious. Your choice to comment on them or to utilize them will depend on your clinical judgment. Below, we provide a brief list of common ideomotor messages.

Examples of Ideomotor Communication

- Blushing
- Blanching
- Darkening around the eyes
- Swallowing

- Muscle tensing
- Other involuntary muscle movements (e.g., leg or foot movements when sitting)
- Tightening fist
- Nodding
- Skin tone
- Posture
- Breathing
- Throat constriction
- Dry mouth
- Voice tone or quality
- Gait
- Eye movements
- Twitching
- Slips of the tongue

DEVELOPMENTAL PROCESSES

Whenever we evaluate our clients for hypnosis and consider which language and images we might use, their age certainly comes into play. Otherwise, we might expect resistance that stems from confusion or ignorance regarding the words that we use. Yet age does not always indicate a client's level of maturation in certain areas. For that reason, we believe it is important to assess our clients as to their functional developmental stage. Without such a consideration, we might encounter unexpected, unconscious agendas that are contrary to our treatment goals.

You might simply ask yourself, "At what age does this client's behavior seem most appropriate?" We are familiar with adults who resort to the temper of a small child or who are preoccupied with the interpersonal drama and need for attention of an adolescent. In designing any therapeutic goal, we know that we must make this developmental age our point of intervention.

Jack was a very worried, overly responsible adult man in the body of a 15-year-old boy. He was brought to my office by his mother because of severe migraine headaches that were causing him to miss school. Yet, with a prematurely furrowed brow, Jack was willing to tell me (RV) that there was a great deal more on his mind. Following his parents' divorce and subsequent financial hardships, he was already preparing for the future. He felt driven to excel in high school, to graduate from a good college, and ultimately to provide for his mother and sister. Although he loved golf, he rarely left himself the time for such recreation.

Meanwhile, Jack's mother was trying to reassure him that they would survive and not to worry. This fell on deaf ears (Jack was quite visual and kinesthetic), as he had already assumed these adult responsibilities. We would need to address both of these competing ego states and their developmental needs: the youthful, playful adolescent and the precocious man of the family.

I asked him to imagine himself on a golf course on a lovely day with a cool breeze. The scene was laid out in great detail as he lined up his shot toward a lush, sloping green. I suggested he have a cool towel around his neck and that he feel the pleasantly chilly breeze blowing. The intent was to relax him while facilitating relief from his headache.

While occasionally checking in on his club selection and perfect reading of the shot he would make, I made suggestions as to how he could best serve his family's needs: that he should be a healthy, happy boy, that he should give his body and mind the time to grow by living in the present, and that he should imagine himself as an adult when he was strong and ready to be his best. Each time we visited this future self, we would then return to the golf course, the cool breeze, and his age-appropriate freedom to be himself. Jack's headache was immediately relieved. We had taped this session so that he could listen to it whenever he felt the first indications of a headache.

This was a situation where a child had assumed an adult ego state. His conflicts were largely conscious and readily accessible. Carla, my (RV) dissociative client previously mentioned, presents a much different picture. In her case, I am treating a grown woman but with several child and adolescent ego states, all of which are either completely dissociated or frequently frightened and mistrusting. One of them is named Shelley.

Carla is a competent, educated woman. Shelley is innocent and shy. Carla tends to be physically demonstrative and even affectionate. Shelley is afraid of touch. Carla wants to move forward, have relationships, and be trusting. Shelley is stuck in time and fearful of men. In order for treatment to be successful, I must respect and address both of their needs. I need to speak openly to Carla while nurturing Shelley's faith in me. Ultimately, we will work to establish a dialogue between them so that Carla can provide for Shelley's growth and development, leading to total integration.

Ideally, normal growth and development flow smoothly and sequentially throughout one's lifetime. One task is successfully completed and our energies are redirected to the next. However, trauma, loss, illness, and a host of other events can interrupt development and arrest maturation. Certain aspects of an individual's functioning remain fixed in time and interfere with age-appropriate functioning. Our clients might have conscious awareness of these unresolved conflicts, but their opportunities for resolution have seemingly passed.

Another analogy to the way in which the unconscious experiences time might be our dreams, where the past, present, and future are often tangled together into some surreal plot. Moreover, in the dream, these odd circumstances will often seem logical. Such is the nature of the unconscious, where we are everyone we have been and, in some respects, everyone we expect to be.

For this reason, we believe hypnosis to be the preferred intervention when developmental issues become the focus of therapy. With access to the distorted realities of the unconscious, we can *dislodge* historical barriers to progress, much like removing a blood clot to improve circulation. In the two clinical examples cited above, we can see how these clients are in some way confused about where they are in time. Jack had progressed to responsibilities beyond his capacities, while Carla can slip into earlier personas depending upon the psychological stressors she encounters.

Through hypnosis, we can assist the conscious and unconscious minds to operate conjointly in the service of the client. With Jack, we externalized his unreasonable adult worries, made explicit his mother's capacity to cope with them, and allowed him to return to age-appropriate responsibilities and activities. Carla is in the process of building better bridges among ego states and learning to trust the adult controlling ego so that they all function more effectively in present time.

Sidney Rosen, MD, in the foreword to Erickson and Rossi's book *The February Man: Evolving Consciousness and Identity in Hypnotherapy* (1989), makes this astute and pertinent observation: "He [Erickson] had the 'child' reenact and abreact to traumatic experiences and, through discussions, guided her through a reeducation process. As a result, the child had new experiences to add to her memories — positive experiences with a caring and understanding adult. These 'corrective regression experiences,' as I have called them, exerted a long-lasting effect on the patient, even after she returned to her adult self."

VIEWING SYMPTOMS AS SOLUTIONS

The unconscious is a marvelously creative yet innocent aspect of the personality. It constantly works to find ways of physically healing, protecting the ego, and helping us to survive and adapt throughout life. The ways in which we learn to adjust to difficulties can initially be productive. However, these adaptations become problematic when dependence on them becomes overgeneralized and/or when they cause difficulties in the client's functioning. In other words, solutions become symptoms. Because the unconscious prefers to perpetuate that which "works," the symptoms themselves are perpetuated and become solutions themselves.

As psychotherapists we must understand that symptoms are not intended to cause the client suffering, as odd as that might sound. One of the amazing things about symptoms is how beautifully they can reflect both the original conflict as well as the unconscious's attempt to correct it. Examples would be the jilted lover who distances from relationships to avoid reinjury or the parents who lose a child and become so emotionally immobilized that they are unable to feel either pain or pleasure. Effective psychotherapy and hypnosis embrace symptoms in this way and work to replace these "solutions" at an unconscious level.

It is sometimes difficult to interpret symptoms in this way. We know that anxiety serves as an alarm to warn of a perceived or internal threat. It is not uncommon for people who fear intimacy to become overweight. Children who are traumatized survive by learning to dissociate. Depression often generates great sympathy and attention. An adolescent's oppositional behavior could be an expression of anger or a developmental need to distance from his parents. Yet why would a 10-year-old boy begin to wet his bed? What would be the advantage of chewing nails or pulling one's own hair out?

As therapists, we do not always need to understand the solution buried in a symptom. In order to truly understand and address the nature of a client's resistance, we need only assume that the solution is inherent in otherwise dysfunctional behavior and give it the respect it demands. We can further assume that the unconscious, in its endeavor to heal all wounds, will accept a healthier alternative behavior when it is offered and proven effective.

You will recall that George had been to numerous psychotherapists, internists, homeopaths, and nutritionists before he called me, yet his symptoms persisted. It would be naïve to think that none of these professionals was capable of helping to relieve his gastric distress and growing aversion to food. Instead, they discovered the extent to which George's symptoms made up a powerful and resilient solution. But to which problem? The answer is found in his family of origin. Food had been his mother's primary means of control and currency of love. The double bind this created for George required a solution, either to become unwittingly enmeshed and compromised by conditional love or to rebel against control. In choosing the latter, he began to refuse his mother's cooking, first voluntarily, and then by developing physiological reactions to food. He became dangerously thin and was eventually hospitalized for depression and anorexia.

By the time George entered my office, the roots and purpose of his distress were no longer conscious to him. Yet his symptoms still sought the same solutions: to have control, to be independent, and to receive attention. Consequently, he was creating a consciously unwanted obstacle to the very help and support that he desperately needed. The alternative solution, then, would be threefold: to develop conscious insight, to build his ego strength and capacity for self-nurturing, and to relieve his gastric symptoms toward a greater desire for feeding. Hypnosis was helpful in the pursuit of these alternative solutions.

CHAPTER 4

Hypnotic Phenomena
and Unconscious Process

ACCESSING UNCONSCIOUS PHENOMENA

At this point, we hope that our readers have begun to place more scrutiny on their client's behavior than on themselves. There is an abundance of information available by viewing much of what a client thinks, feels, says, and does as relevant and useful in hypnotic treatment planning. This broader awareness of behavior and shift in responsibility establishes the groundwork for significantly less performance anxiety and a more natural beginning point for hypnosis.

In chapter 3 we directed your attention specifically to ways of translating everyday characteristics and behavior into a language conducive to hypnosis. We now want to interpret the substance of an individual's healthy and maladaptive functioning as manifestations of his predominant unconscious processes. Our clients enter treatment exhibiting through their waking-state behavior many of the same hypnotic phenomena commonly exploited for trance induction. Symptoms develop when these "talents" have become habituated and problematic. As we begin to recognize the ways in which individuals express such talents through their actions, thoughts, and feelings, a new light is cast on the entire hypnotic progression. When clients are viewed in this way, their unique profiles of hypnotic phenomena suggest a natural conduit through which to begin trance induction and hypnotic treatment planning.

The reader will recognize these phenomena as common means of ratifying trance or for assisting the unconscious to decrease emotional or physical pain. Their normative states are just as familiar but have not yet been identified as such. For example, while we are able to assist someone to become age regressed, many people function in a constant state of age regression. Some adults might be described as playful and others as immature. Both are examples of everyday age regression. Likewise, we have encountered clients who cannot remember the details of their previous session. They experience amnesia, perhaps not only for their therapy but also for other important details of their lives.

We encourage you to identify and utilize these skills instead of ignoring their presence or, worse, attempting to eliminate them. A client who is struggling with the scars of childhood abuse might function in a constant state of age regression and dissociation. Rather than view these symptoms as wholly dysfunctional, we might facilitate age regression to a time prior to the abuse, when the client may have more memories of safety and security. Additionally, we could use her dissociative talents to isolate memories or emotional pain. The same symptom that has served as a dysfunctional "solution" also provides a pathway toward a healthier one.

Marjorie, the hospice nurse mentioned earlier, frequently misplaced her appointment book. More importantly, she would also lose her appointment card, which more directly brought her amnesiac tendencies into therapy. Whereas forgetting the traumas she experienced as a child may have been useful to her survival, in her present life it was leaving her feeling frustrated and incompetent. Through hypnosis, we were able to use this symptom to help her forget about forgetting, thus also using the symptom as part of the solution. In other words, Marjorie already possessed the "skill" of forgetting. Rather than combat that tendency, we used it, paradoxically, to alleviate its overuse.

During trance I asked her unconscious if it would be possible to be more efficient with her ability to forget. Ideomotor signaling indicated that this was acceptable. Using an "apposition of opposites" (Erickson et al., 1976), I said, "You know how to forget and you also know how to forget about forgetting. That is true, is it not?" Ideomotor response indicated "yes." "And now you can learn how to forget only those things that need be forgotten from the past, and can forget to forget the present things you want to know now." Ideomotor response again was "yes." "And this is okay, is it not? To remember what is useful and helpful to know from your present life and to remember to forget only those painful and unnecessary things from the past?" Another ideomotor "yes." "And your unconscious mind knows how to protect you so that when it is useful to remember things in the present, your unconscious and conscious minds can agree to remember. And that, too, is okay, is it not?"

Hypnotic Phenomena

As much as we wish that we had discovered the link between waking-state behavior and hypnotic phenomena, we are only relating the observations and findings of a slew of other teachers and practitioners. When writing about the utilization principle and naturalistic approach to hypnosis, Erickson (1958) wrote, "...the presenting behavior of the patient becomes a definite aid and an actual part in inducing a trance, rather than a possible hindrance (p. 3)." These ideas have been further developed by Brent Geary, PhD (2001a), Stephen Gilligan, PhD (1987), John Edgette, PsyD, and Janet Sasson Edgette, PsyD (1995), among others. We would strongly recommend that our readers further their recognition and comprehension of hypnotic phenomena through the seminars and writings of these teachers to complement the information offered here. However, we believe that this text is somewhat unique in its attempt to translate the hypnotic phenomena present in symptomatic behavior as a means of more readily accessing our clients' hypnotic talents.

The following is a list, with brief descriptions, of commonly occurring hypnotic phenomena that are present in symptomatic behavior and how they can be evoked during trance experiences for therapeutic purposes.

Age regression in everyday life would describe ways in which a person lives in the past. This phenomenon might be manifested as simple immaturity, or be as severe as a preoccupation or an emotional immobility caused by an earlier trauma. In hypnosis, it is the client's ability to experience events from an earlier time in their lives. The revivification of experiences in hypnosis is classified either as partial or whole regressions (Hammond, 1990). "Partial" indicates that the client retains a sense of himself as an adult while remembering events, whereas "full" indicates that the client feels himself to actually be the age that he is remembering. In hypnosis, age regression can be used in a variety of ways. It might be introduced to help a client recall events that have been consciously forgotten or suppressed. It may be used to facilitate pain control, taking the client back to a time before an injury or illness. Likewise, hypnosis could be used to access forgotten abilities or to regress a client to a more functional ego state that existed before experiencing a trauma.

Age progression is essentially the opposite of regression. Typical of someone who is chronically age progressed would be apprehensions about the future or an anticipation of rejection. Using this phenomenon in hypnosis, the client is encouraged to imagine himself in the future. Typically, the purpose of such an intervention is to free the client from her limited view of the present. For a client struggling with a habit control such as overeating or smoking, the therapist might suggest that she could see herself in the future feeling, acting, and thinking in ways that support the changes she desires.

After years of repressing or avoiding emotional pain, whether out of learning or necessity, some individuals become unable to respond to life with the same range as others. In fact, men, who have long been socialized to appear strong and stoic, have been characterized as having normative alexithymia (Levant, 2001). As a hypnotic phenomenon, *anesthesia* is the ability to block the experience of physical or emotional pain. While this might sometimes serve as a beginning point for reintroducing appropriate sensitivities, it would certainly be a skill we can access for the management of acute or chronic discomfort. During surgery or dental procedures, hypnoanesthesia is sometimes the only intervention used by clients. The literature indicates that, at most, only a fifth of the general population is able to create an anesthesia sufficient to serve as the sole anesthetic during medical procedures (Hammond, 1990). More commonly, hypnoanesthesia is combined with pharmacological anesthesia. In psychotherapy, clients who are emotionally very sensitive or have boundaries that are too permeable can benefit from learning to create a degree of emotional anesthesia.

While there is apparently no identified hypnotic phenomenon to describe the antithesis of anesthesia, we might consider the medical term *hypersthesia*, which connotes a heightened sensitivity to physical touch. In psychological terms, we encounter individuals who suffer from emotional *hypersensitivity* (Geary, 2001b). They have become conditioned to react with anger, sadness, or withdrawal to even slight provocation. This is often the case with couples and families who are raw from conflict. Others who experience hypersensitivity are those in early recovery from alcohol or drug dependence who, no longer numbed by self-medication, will recoil from everyday stimuli with acute delicacy.

Amnesia is the complete loss of memory of an event or one's identity. As a naturally occurring hypnotic phenomenon, a person might repress memories or learn to filter the past in advantageous or problematic ways. As a tool in hypnosis, amnesia might be created to lessen the impact of a traumatic situation or to allow the client to forget something that occurred in the hypnotic experience until she is prepared to handle it. For example, sometimes as a person is integrating new material, we can suggest that the client will remember only those things that he currently needs to know at present. Amnesia or selective remembering is used in this case to avoid overwhelming the client.

Hypermnesia, on the other hand, is the ability to remember a representation of the past in great detail. People who are apt to hold grudges might typify this phenomenon in normal living. It might be utilized in hypnosis to enhance memory, perhaps allowing the client to recall helpful details more distinctly or their subjective experience of an event. For example, in forensics, the subject may be encouraged to "zoom in" on a particular aspect of a memory, such as a license plate number or the details of a person's face.

Since trance is itself considered by many to be a state of *dissociation*, it is perhaps the most common naturally occurring hypnotic phenomenon. The "highway hypnosis" described earlier is frequently cited as an example of this split in consciousness. Our traumatized clients often experience spontaneous dissociation in or out of therapy, as they may lose time or their sense of place or of themselves. For these individuals, hypnosis might utilize their talent for dissociation to facilitate a deep trance and work toward eventual reconnecting and integration. Otherwise, this natural talent could be accessed purposely to help clients more effectively distance themselves from painful experiences. For example, it may be used to help clients lessen physical or emotional distress by removing themselves from the experience.

On the other hand, many of our clients have become slaves to their feelings. They suffer day and night, unable to separate themselves from a preoccupation and an enmeshment with their wounds. Once again, this is not an identified hypnotic phenomenon. However, Geary (2001b) has coined the term *association* to identify this state of being overwhelmed with painful affects, cognitions, and/or memories. For example, someone overcome with grief or lost in a blind rage is experiencing the phenomenon of association. As with other hypnotic phenomena, association is a form of focused attention and can be utilized for hypnotic induction. Remember, this *is* the initial goal of the hypnotherapist, not necessarily relaxation.

Psychologically, our clients may experience emotional *catalepsy*, in which they feel "stuck" and unable to move forward with their lives. A client who is experiencing depression, with its accompanying ruminations, hopelessness, and despair, illustrates emotional catalepsy. In hypnosis, catalepsy is the ability to comfortably sustain a certain body posture for extended periods of time. Arm levitation is a common way of inducing catalepsy in hypnosis for the purpose of trance ratification. Clients are often amazed at their ability to remain fixed in a certain position without discomfort. I (MD) had this dramatically illustrated during my visit with Dr. Erickson. He requested I pick up an item he had dropped. As I handed it to him, he placed me in full-body catalepsy. With most of my weight on one foot, I found myself frozen in mid-step.

Others live life in constant flux and confusion, finding it nearly impossible to remain focused on any one thing. These are the clients who incessantly second-guess themselves or find it difficult to prioritize their immediate or long-term goals. Although perhaps at first appearing to be masters at "multitasking," they rarely complete any one objective before becoming distracted by something else. Once again, Brent Geary (2001b) describes this state as *flexibility* or *movement*. We access this talent by hypnotically engaging and pacing this client in a rapidly shifting, multimodal journey through external and internal stimuli, only to lead them toward control and self-containment.

Time distortion refers to the tendency to experience time as either longer (time expansion) or shorter (time condensation) than it actually is. Just about everyone has had the experience of sitting in a boring lecture, feeling as though time is interminable. Conversely, when we are absorbed in an experience, time seems to fly by. Clients who never feel they have enough time experience time condensation, whereas those clients who feel that time cannot pass quickly enough experience time expansion. In hypnosis, clients often experience time distortion without it even being suggested. It happens naturally. As a hypnotic intervention, time expansion can be used to suggest that, while in hypnosis, the client will have all the time necessary to complete the experience. Time condensation is often used with pain control. When

I (MD) worked with a client who had to lie facedown in a headrest as she recovered from an eye surgery, I suggested time condensation to minimize the boredom. She later declared, "I don't know how that works, but it felt as though time went by very quickly."

Positive and negative hallucinations are also common hypnotic phenomena. A positive hallucination occurs when we see something that isn't truly there. While visiting Maine one summer, I (MD) believed there were seals swimming in the harbor. I was convinced that I "saw" a seal's cute face (positive hallucination). With the help of a camera equipped with a zoom lens, I was able to see that these seals were merely bobbing buoys. We still joke about the seals we "saw" that summer. In its more pathological form, the person who irrationally fears that others are plotting to hurt them is experiencing positive hallucinations.

When someone does not see something that is present, this is referred to as a negative hallucination. In its benign form, someone might continually overlook a lost item, only to finally "see" it in its obvious place (negative hallucination). Emotional denial is the failure to acknowledge something that is there because it may be considered too distressing; this could be considered a form of negative hallucination. Clients caught in the cycle of an abusive relationship typically engage in negative hallucinations: They fail to recognize the severity and/or consistency of their abusive experiences.

This utilization of clients' symptoms for their recovery is nicely illustrated in a treatment by Dr. Erickson of a client with phantom limb pain (Erickson et al., 1976). Erickson suggested to the patient that if he could experience phantom limb pain (positive hallucination) in his (missing) foot he could also experience phantom limb pleasure. By expanding upon a skill the patient already possessed, Erickson was able to alleviate the negative symptom by offering a counter example of the same phenomenon.

In addition, Erickson believed that change could best be initiated by targeting a small aspect of a symptom (Haley, 1973). The intent is to create movement and momentum toward change, much like toppling the first of a sequence of dominos. They fall rather slowly with the first few tiles, but gather steam as the action continues. This is very much how hypnosis can initiate change. As Marjorie began remembering important details in her day-to-day life, she was unable to maintain the denial she had been using regarding her present unhappiness. This led to other behavior changes that helped increase her sense of efficacy.

By identifying and utilizing your clients' natural hypnotic abilities, such as I did with Marjorie's amnesia, you not only match the solution to the symptom, but also bypass the resistance that can be encountered by challenging a symptom directly. I accomplished this with Marjorie by suggesting that she "forget about forgetting." Not only was she able to use a skill she already possessed, but she could also do so in a way that allowed her to feel empowered to make other changes. It should be noted that she was not instructed to alter her symptoms, only the way in which she used them. In this approach, we also illustrate to the client the wisdom and adeptness that underlies their symptoms. Symptoms are not random occurrences; rather, they are often in themselves exquisite metaphors for the client's life challenges. By identifying and utilizing them, we show a respect for our clients and the ingenuity of their unconscious in a way that is often overlooked in traditional therapeutic approaches.

The utilization of hypnotic talents can also facilitate a particular outcome in self-hypnosis. A few years ago, I (RV) had to undergo an MRI of my injured shoulder. Not being fond of closed spaces for extended periods of time, I dreaded the ordeal. More specifically, I was anticipating (age progression) that I would not be able to remain calm throughout the eternity (a half-hour) I would be stuck in this machine (time expansion). I knew there would be sounds that might startle me (hypersthesia) and that I would not be able to remain still and calm (a fear of catalepsy). Given the strength of my expectations, I decided not to avoid these stressors, but to utilize them in a self-hypnotic experience. I took myself to my favorite North Carolina beach and *looked forward* to a *long*, relaxing day *lying still* in the sun. I paid *close attention* to the MRI air conditioner that had become a cool ocean breeze. The nurse's voice and loud noises became the irritating but *familiar distractions* of a rude family behind me. Given a less-than-perfect situation, I created a less-than-perfect fantasy by utilizing my predominant hypnotic phenomena (age progression, hypersthesia, and catalepsy) at the time.

Table 4.1 demonstrates the presence of hypnotic phenomena in normal, problematic, and pathological functioning.

TRANCE DEPTH AND BREADTH

Trance Depth

The scientists in our profession would almost certainly groan at the suggestion that trance depth is not always important. We understand

Table 4.1

Hypnotic phenomenon	Normal behavior	Problematic behavior	Dysfunctional behavior
Age regression	Playfulness Curiosity	Impulsiveness Temper	Dependence Immaturity
Age progression	Foresight Fantasizing	Worry Procrastination	Immobilizing fear Avoidance
Amnesia	Misplacing Tip of the tongue	Forgetfulness	Repressed memories
Hypermnesia	Good memory Attention to detail	Grudges Rumination	Abreaction Obsessive ritual
Anesthesia	High pain tolerance	Emotionally closed	Depression
Hypersensitivity (hypersthesia)	Emotionally sensitive Rumination	Defensiveness Vigilance Feeling slighted	Emotionally overwhelmed Paranoia
Time condensation	Time flying by	Chronic lateness	Loss of time
Time expansion	Time passing by slowly	Feeling a bad situation will never end	Hopelessness Despair
Dissociation	Avoiding feelings	Emotional numbing	Multiple personality Eating disorders
Association	Preoccupation	Emotionally or cognitively flooded	Flashbacks Immobilized
Catalepsy	Frustration	Feeling "stuck"	Rigidly avoiding change
Flexibility	Flighty Indecisive	Continually distracted Lacking foresight	Hysteria

that the hallmarks of various depths of trance have been studied and well documented (Watkins, 1987; Weitzenhoffer, 1989). Tools have been developed to demonstrate an individual's hypnotizability and are taught in most beginning hypnosis trainings (Shor & Orne, 1962;

Spiegel & Spiegel, 1978; Weitzenhoffer & Hilgard, 1959). Such measurements would certainly be helpful in research on how the effectiveness of hypnosis in various settings and situations would be related to the talents of the subjects involved. Clinically speaking, greater trance depth might be helpful in accessing early life experience or facilitating a change in deeply entrenched belief systems. Theoretically, the deeper the trance, the more unconscious processes will be accessible to suggestion (Erickson et al., 1976; Weitzenhoffer, 1989).

Facilitating Trance Depth
It is likely, however, that concern about creating greater trance depth will only raise unnecessary anxiety for the hypnotherapist. If a deep trance is assumed to be the responsibility of the clinician and an indication of successful hypnosis, therapists might become inhibited from developing their skills. When you have learned to read and utilize predictable physiological, emotional, and hypnotic phenomena, you will find that trance depth is more easily facilitated by your own powers of observation. As you recognize and incorporate your clients' unique talents as part of your induction, their absorption will become greater.

Many beginning hypnotherapists persevere with suggestions for relaxation as a means of deepening trance. However, this preoccupation can often prove to be counterproductive with certain clients, as it establishes a premise that is contrary to what we know about trance. This is not to say that relaxation and calming imagery are not beneficial in many hypnotic protocols. Yet if a person who is merely driving in traffic can be in trance, then relaxation is obviously not the least bit necessary to becoming deeply hypnotized. The revivification of painful traumatic memories during an abreaction would evoke conditions that are the antithesis of relaxation. In treatment we will sometimes suggest anxiety symptoms in order to demonstrate a client's unconscious talents, only to then reduce the intensity of her symptoms. We can see how such expectations are truly unrealistic in working with children, who will often fidget, scratch, and even talk during significantly deep trance.

Most hypnotherapists attempt to facilitate trance depth through suggestions of increasing absorption. We "attach" deeper relaxation to taking breaths, counting numbers, walking down steps, or watching clouds pass by. Just about any experience can be used as an attachment for progressive deepening of trance. With this method, the progressive deepening of trance can be facilitated by a myriad of attachments that may be of the therapist's making or fashioned from imagery known to be favored by the client. This is a very common method of deepening and has been the cornerstone of many traditional hypnotic inductions. However, this can be experienced as a bit artificial, as the client must incorporate imagery suggested by the therapist to deepen his own trance experience. In contrast, a naturalistic approach utilizing the client's nonverbal behaviors and experiences reflects his intrinsic hypnotic abilities and can thus feel more natural and spontaneous.

This point was highlighted to us during the authors' first encounter, when we both attended an ASCH Individualized Consultation workshop. Marc Oster, PsyD, suggested that I (MD) demonstrate a naturalistic induction for the benefit of other participants who were less familiar with this approach. Each of them reported feeling that their trance state was more vivid, natural and dramatic than their typical experiences of trance.

Depths of Trance

While we do not want to contradict ourselves or encourage performance anxiety in our readers, we would be remiss if we didn't review the recognizable depths of trance (Hammond, 1988).

Hypnoidal (light) trance. The client begins to look as though she is in a state beyond relaxation. The client is in rapport with the therapist and feels a sense of safety. This state is characterized by a fluttering of the eyelids, an inability to open the eyes, deep, slow breathing, and physical relaxation and feelings of muscular lethargy. She may look asleep but, because of her posture and responsiveness to the therapist's suggestions, she is not. We might be familiar with this level of trance as that feeling we have when we daydream. Our general reality orientation is muted and distant as our breathing slows and movement is limited. Our hypnotically experienced clients sometimes enter this level of trance prior to the introduction of formal induction techniques.

Medium trance. This state is not easily discernible without using specific tests to evaluate its presence. These tests might include the client's ability to produce such phenomena as glove anesthesia, partial amnesia, or hallucinations. Clients tend to be aware of their physical surroundings but are no longer compelled to respond.

Deep trance (somnambulism). In this state of trance, as in sleep, self-reflective awareness is not present. Hypnotic tests can demonstrate

somnambulism by assessing the client's ability to open his eyes without affecting the trance *or* to experience extensive anesthesia, age
regression, and/or lip pallor.

Plenary trance (stuporous).   This depth of trance will most likely seldom occur in your everyday practice of hypnosis. Your client loses his
awareness of time, body, and the external world. His heart rate and
breathing drop off considerably as the mind and body disconnect from
any need to remain alert or aroused for spontaneous thought or action.

Depth through Breadth

In an effort to identify the process by which we utilize unconscious
process toward the facilitation of trance depth, we suggest the concept
of *breadth* of trance experiences. In the previous section, we discussed
the hypnotic phenomena implied by our clients' presentations. These
idiosyncratic "talents" establish a beginning point for hypnosis that,
when accessed, will contribute to a broader focused absorption and
utilization of one's unconscious.

Consider Matthew, a 30-year-old research assistant who complained of generalized anxiety, hypersensitivity to criticism, and a life
paralyzed by both. Hypnotically, he could be described as cataleptic,
hypersensitive (Geary, 2001b), and experiencing both positive hallucinations and time condensation. With an excessive need for control,
he would also be highly resistant yet quite motivated for relief. Given
this profile, I (RV) opted for a direct induction to utilize his enthusiasm,
but with permissive, confusional language to bypass conscious
resistance.

His focus in hypnosis, however, would be the hypnotic phenomena already present. I safely predicted the tensing of his muscles, his
intrusively racing thoughts, a sense of temporal immediacy, and freez-
ing of affective experience. It was not difficult to absorb him in his
own experience, and he was readily brought to a moderate depth of
trance. I predicted that, as he continued to follow these thoughts and
note the tension in his shoulders and face, he would find it easier to
progress to an even deeper trance. He was "allowed" to increase these
symptoms slightly as a means of both retaining control and of ratifying
his trance experience. Once he "accepted responsibility" for his experience, I was then able to lead him gradually into a comfortably relaxed
state ("acceptable to you at this time," of course).

By not owning the responsibility for his depth of trance and by engaging him in his own hypnotic phenomena, I was, in essence, utilizing his "breadth" of trance to create depth. Once he gained confidence in his skills of entering trance and understood there was no surrendering of his own controls, we were able to begin further hypnotic work in a more trusting and cooperative way.

We believe that trance breadth can be more naturally produced through the accurate utilization of natural and hypnotic phenomena. The premise, again, is that our clients are already presenting with characteristic hypnotic skills. Matthew was frequently in a state of catalepsy, hypersthesia, positive hallucination, and time condensation and had an excessive need for control. My intent was to utilize these "skills" by absorbing him in them. Had I sought to engage him in immediate relaxation or metaphors for safety, I would have been working against his tendencies and trance depth would have been more difficult to achieve.

Instead, we helped him to enter trance through the doors that were already slightly ajar. He was ready and willing to be hypervigilant, tense, and anxious. Mirroring these tendencies in the induction allowed the client to feel safe, since I was only asking him to do what he was already doing. In other words, going into a trance felt congruent with his experience as opposed to something that felt foreign or forced. With this method, one achieves the additional benefits of trance ratification and the enhancement of trust in the hypnotic relationship.

In our clinical experience, we find that the subjective experience of trance is different when induced by naturalistic rather than directive techniques. Client reports indicate that a naturalistic trance approach feels more congruent. We believe this enhances the client's sense of ownership of the hypnotic experience. Directive trance experiences can be experienced as slightly alien, with the client feeling more of a demand to perform in a certain way that may not be natural to them. Although both methods are effective, the paths to trance depth in these two styles take a slightly different course.

"Breadths" of Trance

As we have shown earlier, there are levels of trance depth that are generally recognized through observation as well as formal assessments. We propose that there might also be stages or levels of trance "breadth." They are meant to capture a subjective continuum that originates with a client's existing unconscious process. Greater trance breadth is then achieved through increasing degrees of absorption and focus. The levels are:

"Preconscious hypnotic talent."   This describes the idiosyncratic hypnotic phenomena through which an individual enters regularly occurring trance states. These are waking-state manifestations of hypnotic phenomena that are characteristic of both healthy and unhealthy functioning. For example, when we are deeply absorbed in a task, we are naturally using dissociation or experiencing negative hallucinations, that is, ignoring distracting stimuli. Conversely, when the anxious person becomes absorbed in his racing heart and shortness of breath, he is, in effect, in a trance state (hypermnesia). The depressed person is overwhelmed by the seemingly endless night and is, in a sense, in trance (time expansion).

"Self-absorption."   Through therapeutic, naturalistic utilization of predictable talents and subjective experience, the individual enters trance as he establishes focus and absorption into his preconscious talents. Thus, when we ask our clients to attend to what is presently occurring, be it the rhythm of their breathing or their racing thoughts, we are employing their subjective experience as a means to engage them hypnotically. These naturally occurring phenomena can thus become the path along which a "broader" trance experience is attained. We merely guide them in taking the additional steps along the path to a greater level of hypnotic involvement.

"Self-surrender."   The individual yields to a deeper trance experience through an unconscious reconciliation between adaptive, self-protective resistance and her safely familiar hypnotic phenomena. By emphasizing a congruency between what she is already experiencing and what is possible or likely, the client is able to further her trance experience. At this level of breadth, her defenses are minimized, thus allowing her to achieve a sufficient degree of suggestibility and attention to trance experience.

"Hypnotic synchronicity."   The client becomes more absorbed in his unconscious process and can access and affect healthy or maladaptive manifestations of hypnotic phenomena. This is a level of trance breadth at which very deep internal work becomes possible. As the individual becomes immersed in the hypnotic experience, boundaries to awareness and imagination fade. The client is no longer bound by

the typical limits of logical thinking as "trance logic" (Erickson et al., 1976) and possibilities open up potentials for change that logical approaches cannot allow.

Our readers might conclude that the distinction between trance depth and breadth is merely semantic. In truth, we might agree. Both terms are, after all, hypothetical constructs invented to describe a subjective experience. The distinction has less to do with actual trance experience than it does with the means of accessing that experience. We merely wish to remind you that your clients have inherent hypnotic abilities that can be both utilized and emphasized for the induction of trance. This view requires you to sharpen your observational skills, your knowledge of human physiology, and your familiarity with your client. Your reward is that the induction of hypnosis and utilization of trance will become more fluid and effortless. Furthermore, there will be a greater appreciation for the client's potentials and more realistic expectations for the role of hypnotist.

CHAPTER 5

Treatment Planning: Accessing Natural Trance

THE LANGUAGE OF HYPNOTIC INDUCTION

As I (RV) supervised Joan during a small group hypnotherapy practice, she stumbled over her words, turned to me, and whispered, "I think I need help here." Her client was comfortably in trance, paying no attention to her panicked aside to me. Upon observing her apparently successful work thus far, I simply said, "No you don't." She looked stunned at first and then proceeded.

Until that point, I had paid little attention to her words. What struck me about her induction was the graceful flow of her arms and hands. She was like an orchestra conductor enrapt by a lovely adagio. Without her noticing, her movements had become the focal point of her hypnotic language, not her words. Even after her subject's eyes had closed, she continued to "speak" in her own unique way. Once given permission to rely on her strengths, she relaxed and her confidence began to blossom.

Too many hypnotherapists, both beginning and advanced, become overly concerned about words. They soften their voices and struggle to "make" their clients relax. Assuming the full responsibility for such an impossible assignment, they become preoccupied and self-conscious with their words. While there certainly are recommended ways of structuring hypnotic language toward specific applications, these are only guidelines that must be adapted to one's own communication style. There really is no one preferred path to trance induction. Like a dancer watching her own feet, a hypnotherapist who is focused on her own performance will likely stumble over herself in an attempt to speak in just the "right" way. By doing so, she becomes blinded to the true source of effective hypnotic language sitting across from her.

Even for clients who have been previously hypnotized, each trance experience is unique. Until she knows her client well, a psychotherapist will have more success by approaching hypnosis as an experiment with no set expectations. In her own words, she reflects her client's present physical, emotional, and cognitive status as a point of entry. With the practice of mirroring and accurate feedback, there is no effort to change any facet of this presentation. She speaks the truths that she witnesses and those she knows about human functioning. When unsure of what to say next, she utilizes the silence and promotes some vague unconscious choice her client might be making. The question you might ask yourself at this point is not, "Am I using the correct language?," but "Am I helping my client to create an internal focused absorption?" The latter, with the possible addition of a trance ratification experience, is the sole purpose of the hypnotic induction. Even the possible confusion caused by an extended silence or a misspoken phrase can contribute toward this intent.

When in doubt, pass the ball back to your clients where it belongs. Given what we know about our clients' ability to project meaning and distort messages (positive hallucination), we assign responsibility for the correct language to them. For example, consider the words of Joseph Barber, PhD (Hammond & Cheek, 1988), when he says, "And since I can't really know exactly the things that you need to hear right now, I hope that you will listen to your unconscious mind, because you have the ability to automatically create the words that you need to hear — an ability to automatically hear the words that you most want."

Choosing a Path

Perhaps it would be helpful to think of the hypnotic induction as more of a conversation than a monologue. Your client speaks to you through the numerous facets of his presentation, and you then respond to all of this information through words, tone, posture, and pacing. Even with a formal, more direct induction, you can enhance the shared trance experience by allowing your words to be tailored by what you receive from the person before you.

We believe the distinction among naturalistic, indirect, and direct induction to be largely artificial. There can and should be elements of all three incorporated into your language, with the emphasis determined by individual client differences. The language of utilization will promote an unconscious bond between you and your client and bypass resistance. Indirect, permissive language ensures success and builds momentum toward trance ratification and feelings of empowerment. It manages to seed helpful suggestions that can bypass conscious resistance while assisting the client to have more direct access to her unconscious resources. Direct language, used selectively, reinforces the influence of the hypnotherapist, which will later enhance post-hypnotic suggestion. The highly motivated and trusting client might prove to be more suggestible and would thus benefit from a more directive and authoritative hypnotic style. As with Joan, all of this is held together by your personality and style.

In chapter 4 we discussed the translation of normal and symptomatic behavior into terms of hypnotic phenomena. We consider these behaviors to be clues to knowing where to begin and what to say. You will essentially be "going with the grain," so to speak. For example, I (RV) routinely use an induction that features dissociation (arm levitation, Chaisson, hand magnets) with a client whose behavior suggests dissociation (compulsive eating, dissociative identity disorder). I will involve an anxious client (age progression, hypermnesia) in a somewhat frenetic fantasy of rapidly changing future and past images while calling attention to muscle tension and control. Does this encourage relaxation? No. Does it lead my client into a focused absorption? Yes.

The anxious client with shortness of breath and chest palpitations is in trance. The dissociative client is in trance as she reexperiences a childhood ego state (Edgette & Edgette, 1995; Gilligan, 1987; Lankton & Lankton, 1983). The burn victim in the emergency room, consumed by constant pain and fear, is in trance (Hammond, 1990). An individual does not have to be relaxed to be in trance. That is not your initial goal. Your goal is to assist your client in reaching a state of focused absorption. That is the purpose of induction. From that point, you can then redirect him toward containment and a vivid experience of increasing strength and control.

In even broader terms, we might consider the states of consciousness in which trance most commonly occurs. If we believe that consciousness lies on a continuum, then trance states would probably occur at either end (see Figure 5.1 below).

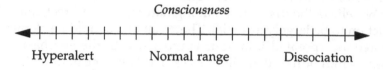

Consciousness

Hyperalert   Normal range   Dissociation

Figure 5.1

On one end of this continuum would be hyperalertness, with dissociation at the other. In the center are more usual waking states that reflect alertness to some aspects of one's experience and dissociation from others. Whether a person is hyperalert and experiencing (anxiety, rage, performing) or is completely detached and dissociated from the outside world (daydreaming, emotionally flat), he is in a very absorbed, pre-hypnotic state. We can guide our clients into trance by understanding and utilizing their normal tendencies toward either extreme. In other words, if he is the kind of person whose mind tends to wander or disengage from his surroundings, we would offer imagery that promotes detachment. For example, "As you hear my voice, you can also rest in the knowledge that there is nothing that you have to do right now; nowhere to go, nowhere to be, just time to be; letting go of anything unnecessary." Conversely, if he is more likely to enter trance states through hypervigilance or anxiety, you would encourage his attention even to those symptoms from which he wants to be relieved, e.g., the pounding of his heart or his endless intellectualizations and obsessions.

Remember that the hypnotic induction is not only intended to create trance, but also to confirm your client's capacity to utilize his unconscious for growth and healing. Trance ratification, as it is called, involves a demonstration of hypnotic phenomena for the purpose of making your client a believer (Weitzenhoffer, 1989). During an advanced workshop demonstration, my (RV) volunteer subject asked for help with appetite control. He was obese and reported that his problem was frequent "unconscious eating." When asked what type of induction he wanted to be demonstrated, he requested an arm levitation. Knowing that his eating disorder reflected a talent for dissociation and that his stated preference would positively influence his expectations, I consented and the levitation was successful. My next step was to use my subject's talent to reinforce his confidence. It was suggested that, as the balloon lost air and his arm fell gently to his lap, his unconscious mind would find ways to solve his dilemma and that his awareness of hunger and fullness would make a permanent correction. When the arm levitates or the eyes close involuntarily, the power of the unconscious has been validated and many barriers to future hypnotic work and change have been diminished.

NATURALISTIC UTILIZATION

As I (RV) was leaving the theater after seeing the movie *Magnolia* (1999), I said aloud to no one in particular, "What the hell was that?" followed soon after by, "Wow, that was terrific!" After multiple viewings, I am not sure I fully understand this film, but it has become one of my favorites. I recall when, as a beginning hypnotherapist, I heard utilization language as both confusing and lovely. It was like hearing the beautiful words of classic poetry, whose meaning remained elusive. In my first hypnotic experience many years ago, I was led into a deep and peaceful trance while having no idea how this had been achieved. Later, in my beginning class, we learned a "cookbook" method of hypnosis: first, the choice of rather mechanical inductions, then the deepening language, and finally a few direct post-hypnotic suggestions. With the exception of an emphasis on permissive language, we were given the distinct impression that we were responsible for our client's trance. I had learned the skills, but had not yet learned the language.

What made naturalistic language seem so difficult to grasp was that it seemed so very spontaneous and benign. I was afraid that this was a skill that only those who had been immersed in hypnosis for ages could master. There seemed to be no technique, no uniform rhythm, no edge, and no script. My fears were primarily based on the beginner's false premise as to who is responsible for the trance. It is not the therapist who must find the right words. The therapist places her focus on her client, who will guide him to the right words. As with the relationship between a musician and his guitar, it is the instrument that emits a sound but it is the player who must learn how to evoke the range and depth of sound that his instrument can create.

Naturalistic induction refers to the selection of appropriate language to access, observe, and utilize clients' voluntary and involuntary behavior, adaptive resistance, and unconscious process. What was once elusive about this language has become so very obvious. Words that seem so simplistic — to comment on shifts in posture, swallowing, breathing, or a brief scan of what I know to be true about an internal focus — are so powerful when heard with the correct timing and delivery.

One critical value to naturalistic language is its ability to bypass conscious thought and resistance. By observing and predicting indisputable facts about human functioning and your client's idiosyncratic behavior, resistance erodes and the client's attention and interest in your words increases. Because they are indisputable statements of fact, these "truisms" of human behavior are irresistible to the unconscious. Feelings of recognition and understanding allow apprehension and mistrust to soften. Doors begin to open.

We can gain an even greater advantage by speaking truisms that also reflect the person's predominant sensory style. The following are a few examples:

Visual
- "Throughout your life you have seen some things and not seen some things that you could have seen if you paid attention to them."
- "As you focus on that spot, the light around it may change and vary from time to time..."

Auditory
- "As you hear my voice, the voice of your own thoughts will come in and out..."
- "Sometimes you will hear my words and sometimes you might hear the sounds around you."

Kinesthetic
- "You can feel your hands resting comfortably on your lap."
- "Your breathing will continue in its own natural rhythm, just as with each exhale, you can let go of more and more unnecessary tension..."

Below are the hallmarks of naturalistic induction that can be helpful in framing suggestions. The list is inherently incomplete as the potential for truisms or observable behavior is virtually endless.

Elements of Naturalistic Inductions

- Observation and prediction of noticeable bodily process — external
    Breathing and pacing
    Blinking and fluttering
    Swallowing
    Facial tone
    Changes in skin color
    Muscle tension
- Observation and prediction of presumable bodily process — internal
    Breathing — rate, sound, feel
    Heartbeat, pulse
    "Internal eyes"
    Lightness/heaviness
    What can be "seen" with closed eyes
    Areas of tension and relaxation
- Observation and prediction of normal mental activity
    Internal dialogue
    Attention to external sounds
    Listening/not listening
    Holding on/letting go
- Creating an internal focus
    How they anticipate the trance experience to be
    Remembering times when they might have experienced trance
    Suggestions for a sensory experience of familiar places or people
    Progressive muscle tensing and relaxation
- Attention to sensory strengths and interests
    Using visual, auditory, or tactile language that reflects client
        strength
    Suggestions for imagery that reflects client's work and pre-
        ferred activities

Should all this still sound too complicated, it isn't. But there is one sensory experience that you can be certain your client is experiencing: her breath. Erickson believed that matching your client's breathing with your own could best facilitate rapport as well as trance induction. We believe that, by pacing your suggestions with the client's inhalations and exhalations, they will seem more like a part of a natural process.

INDIRECT AND DIRECT LANGUAGE

Indirect Language

The use of permissive, indirect language appeals to an innate need and wish to be the architect of our own existence. From a young age we bridle at being told what to do or forced into doing anything, even for our "own good." In choosing, we exert our will and direct our course. The suggestion of hypnosis, with the common misconception that it involves a loss of control, almost invariably invites resistance. The use of indirect and permissive language helps to circumvent this resistance. Its use allows the client to choose not only whether she will respond, but *how.* The therapist offers the client a host of alternatives through ambiguous suggestions. The client is given the freedom to refuse one alternative, while pondering or choosing the other. As I (RV) am often quoting Yogi Berra to my clients, "When you come to a fork in the road, take it!" (Berra, Kaplan, & Kaplan, 2001).

Permissive language feels "soft" to the ear and to the psyche. It is, in essence, also more respectful of the client in that it assumes that the client will choose in a way that is in service of her development. Rather than being told, "You will...," the client accurately perceives that he is in charge with words such as "perhaps," "you might," "maybe," and, of course, "I really don't know." These words encourage the client's unconscious to seek its own answers rather than rely upon the therapist to be the expert.

The following is a list of typical features of permissive and indirect induction styles.

Elements of Indirect Inductions

- Permissive language
- Dissociative language
- Predicting the inevitable (truisms)
- Abstract hypnoprojectives
- Open post-hypnotic suggestions
- Confusion techniques to bypass conscious thought, e.g., conscious/unconscious double binds
- Pacing and leading
- Use of metaphor
- Paradoxical directives
- Use of presuppositions

Direct Language

We propose that any hypnotic induction should include naturalistic and permissive language, for the reasons cited above. However, the use of a more authoritative style is sometimes preferable, such as when working with highly hypnotizable, trusting, or motivated clients. Likewise, clients who are in the midst of a medical crisis, such as a burn or accident victim, are highly motivated, easily accessible, and find direct suggestions grounding. Powerful, ego-enhancing direct suggestions can even help to nudge a depressed client out of his cataleptic inertia or to contain the individual who is lost in a morass of conflicting emotions and thoughts. Because direct language offers the potential for a more rapid constructive response, opportunities for its use should not be missed.

Jennifer, a newly married young woman, came to treatment because she was sexually unresponsive to her husband. Both she and her spouse interpreted this as meaning that she did not find him desirable. Yet Jennifer claimed that desire was not her issue. Rather, she believed that her difficulties with arousal were rooted in her childhood when she was taught that, to remain "pure," she could not allow herself to enjoy herself sexually. Believing that Jennifer needed permission to become responsive, I (MD) made the error of using permissive language in our initial trance work. As a former supervisor once warned me, "When you get it wrong, your client will tell you one way or the other, over and over if necessary, what they need." When Jennifer came out of her trance, she protested, "But you didn't tell me what to do!" She had expected and wanted direct suggestions in order to overcome her long-standing internalized directives from childhood.

Jennifer is a good example of a client who offers little resistance to direct suggestion. Because I had not accurately assessed her expectations for hypnosis and immediate faith in me, I misread the role that she had hoped I would take. She had wanted a firm but nurturing expert to replace an obsolete belief system with one more consistent with her adult stage of development. In a few short sessions with "the doctor," Jennifer overcame her sexual arousal disorder.

The trust and positive expectations requisite to using direct suggestions can be either immediately present or developed through rapport-building and trance-ratification methods. Ideally, all clients would be responsive to an authoritative style so that the hypnotherapist could exert more influence toward positive change. Therefore,

any and all efforts to cultivate a solid, cooperative hypnotic relationship will be rewarded with greater efficiency and success.

Following are some of the hallmarks of direct inductions:

Elements of Direct Induction

- Authoritative language
- Concrete predictions of hypnotic phenomena
- Simple, declarative affirmations
- Prescribing solutions
- Tending to be more dramatically trance-ratifying
- Useful in assessing the effectiveness of post-hypnotic suggestions
- Most effective with clients who are:
  - trusting/low resistance
  - motivated
  - have positive expectations for hypnosis
  - highly hypnotizable
  - in an urgent state

PREPARING FOR HYPNOTIC WORK: "TO SCRIPT OR NOT TO SCRIPT"

We can assume that most writers are avid readers. Musicians and
composers study and imitate the works of their predecessors and
contemporaries. Dancers are taught moves named for the great cho-
reographers. Why, then, should psychotherapists not benefit from the
valuable and innovative language found in hypnotic scripts? We
strongly encourage you to read and reread others' scripts even if you
decide not to use them in treatment. When you do choose to read them
in therapy, you can do so somewhat surreptitiously or completely
openly. My (RV) method was to conduct one of the formal inductions
I had learned in basic training and, when my client's eyes were closed,
I would take my glasses and script from my desk and wax eloquent
with borrowed material. Other times, I would simply inform my client
that I had a "special procedure that would be particularly helpful" to
him and read from the script openly.

I (RV) informed one particularly tense and apprehensive client
that I was in possession of a very interesting and humorous script and
offered to share it with him. I was referring to a page of confusional
language I had received from Norma and Phil Barretta at a recent
workshop. As I slowly read to him, he became very still and his eyes

began to flutter. Without missing a beat, I launched into suggestions of control, safety, and peace. In future sessions, he sometimes asked me to "try out" more of this interesting language. Thus, from the words of others, a successful hypnotic intervention was born.

While scripts will help you to learn and gain some level of confidence with hypnotic language, we advise that you eventually integrate others' words into your own style and powers of observation. When I (MD) first read *Hypnotic Realities* (1976), by Erickson, Rossi, and Rossi, I wondered if I would ever fully understand, much less apply, what these legends were talking about. However, after several readings, I began to memorize entire passages from Erickson's inductions to use as scripts. After all, they were filled with masterful permissive and indirect nuggets that would fit for almost any client. Many of their words have found their way into my usual hypnotic language and have certainly served as an inspiration in helping me to gain confidence in my own ideas and talent for observation.

Writing "customized" scripts for certain clients can be useful in meeting their individual needs. Their unique characteristics, sensory strengths, and potential for resistance can be more easily addressed. This practice will also facilitate the hypnotist's familiarity and comfort with his own metaphors.

Cliff was a graduate student who was struck by a drunk driver and became a paraplegic at age 17. He began therapy when he could not finish his dissertation. Bound to a wheelchair for much of his life, he had pursued an education against incredible odds. Cliff hated his disability and felt it robbed him of a normal life. He felt ashamed of needing a wheelchair and bristled at anyone who tried to help him or who commented in any way about his illness. His resentment was enormous. Being extremely bright and verbal, Cliff's sarcasm could be razor sharp, leaving the recipient speechless. I (MD) often found myself sympathizing with the uninitiated who might trespass into Cliff's psychological space.

Cliff appeared to be as frustrated with his dissertation stalemate as he was with his disability. In both cases, he was stuck (or "cataleptic"). Aware that his frustration was immense and that he had entered therapy as reluctantly as he used his wheelchair, I knew that I needed to proceed cautiously with Cliff. He, like many disabled people, faced incredible physical frustrations every day of his life. I felt that I had to be careful not to humiliate him with further failure (negative hallucination), while also not becoming immobilized or intimidated by his potential for volatility.

I realized that Cliff was in a double bind. He feared that, if he finished his dissertation and moved on with his life, the man who had severely altered his life would somehow be vindicated. Cliff believed that his success would "let that s.o.b. off the hook for hurting me." However, the inability to complete his dissertation would continue to empower his enemy as well and would perpetuate his role of helpless victim.

I felt that I needed to be very clear about what I wanted to suggest to Cliff, as I could easily err on one side or the other of his dilemma. To do so could easily evoke anger and/or mistrust that would lead to resistance to all suggestions. I chose to write scripts for our hypnotic work as a way to navigate through the complexities and potential therapeutic hazards of Cliff's situation. I decided to build my script on a pacing and leading model with the intention of establishing a "yes" set as the groundwork for an acceptance of new ideas. With Cliff, it was extremely important to enter his emotional space by "pacing" with his intense anger and resentment (hypersthesia, age regression) that contributed to his emotional entrenchment (catalepsy). Next, it would be necessary to "lead" by suggesting alternatives that would produce forward movement and healing. Cliff's script included the following statements:

> "And you know how to feel disappointed..." (pacing)
> "You know the experience of wondering if anything will ever be any better..." (pacing)
> "You sometimes see few choices for happiness..." (pacing)
> "And you really don't know when or how any or all of those experiences will change in the future..." (leading)
> "You really wonder how your mind or spirit will help you to become free in every possible way open to you..." (leading)
> "You really don't know when you will secure a foothold in your own future..." (leading)
> "Or how you will reclaim your energy and intelligence...to leave that 's.o.b.' in the dust..." (leading)

Cliff was caught between his desires to have a rewarding life and his vengeful wish to punish the person who had hurt him. So my script needed to carefully capture and validate both of these aspects. In choosing to use pacing and leading suggestions, I could mirror the client's emotional tone as well as the paradoxical conflict inherent in his dilemma. As is evident, my pacing suggestions reflected what already existed for Cliff, while my leading suggestions implied a direction toward which he might move. The added benefit of accommodating my client's paradox was to discharge the emotional undertone that has immobilized him. The advantage of preparing his script was to incorporate all that I wanted to say while avoiding the potential for resistance created by his predicament.

DEEPENING LANGUAGE AND NONVERBAL CUES

In the 1931 black-and-white film *Svengali*, John Barrymore brings to life a very sinister version of the title character. As he leans closely over an innocent young woman, he eerily commands, "You are going deeper, deeper, deeper, Lichen." With a frightening, menacing presence, his eyes glow a deep red as he whispers, "You will think only of Svengali, Svengali!" Entranced by his power, she breathes, "Svengali..." In triumph, he hisses, "Yessss! Svengali!"

This stereotypical authoritarian portrayal of hypnosis reinforces the myth that trance depth is correlated to the optimal hypnotic experience and that the subject is under the hypnotist's control. We believe that depth is often not necessary in achieving our hypnotherapeutic goals. Rather than seeking greater depth, we prefer to utilize the breadth of uniquely individual hypnotic talents that clients present.

The achievement of a greater "breadth" of trance is an extension of the same hypnotic language as used in the induction process. Instead of thinking of deepening as the second stage of hypnosis, we prefer to think of hypnosis as a continuum of breadth and depth. Once your client exhibits trance behavior, you simply continue to suggest greater absorption in the experience. We learn techniques such as walking down stairs (noticing the texture of the carpet and the wood grain of the banister) or riding in an elevator "down...down." The value in these exercises is that they continue to facilitate greater focus and absorption in the trance experience.

The suggestion of greater absorption and depth can also be attached to the internal or external experience of the client. Virtually any stimulus can be utilized for this purpose. For example, I (RV) routinely suggest to my clients that "any sounds or distractions that might occur will only take you deeper into this pleasant experience." Most often, it is preferable to attach the client's internal focus, and subsequent depth, to images familiar and comfortable for him.

For example, John, a depressed client, entered therapy because his physical symptoms were ruled out as being physically based. His most distressing physical symptom, pain around his heart, appeared to be metaphorical for the heartache he was feeling over the loss of his marriage. It is not difficult to see that John's primary sensory system was tactile. He couldn't help but "feel" things to their utmost. Likewise, John was a biking enthusiast and was well aware that on his long rides he could dissociate from physical pain.

John's talents for being tactilely sensitive as well as his ability to create a pleasant physical dissociation were utilized to enhance his trance experience. John was already struggling with the depths of depression; he did not need to go deeper! My suggestions focused upon "letting go" and allowing himself to recreate a pleasant dissociation from emotional pain by "going further" into his trance experience.

Likewise, John had learned to modulate his breathing to sustain stressful exertion during his bike rides. While in trance his slowed breath was likened to slowing down and better tolerating the stress of dealing with loss. A slower breathing pattern is typical of many trance experiences and can be utilized both to enhance the trance experience itself and for clients overwhelmed with either anxiety or depression as a cue to slow down and take one thing at a time.

CHAPTER 6

Treatment Planning: Resistance and the Metaphor

MANAGING AND UTILIZING RESISTANCE: DISRUPTING RIGID/CONSCIOUS SETS

Resistance is essentially adaptive, self-protective behavior (Lankton & Lankton, 1983; Yapko, 1995). It represents an effort to ward off threats to the familiar reality regardless of how unhealthy that might be. Consequently, these defenses usually present a most durable and tenacious unconscious barrier to change. Psychotherapists fear resistance because it will potentially derail their efforts and threaten their feelings of competence. Meanwhile, our clients are unwittingly caught in a form of psychological prison which they are reluctant to leave.

As with symptoms, resistance is a solution. Indeed, resistance is usually a manifestation of predominant hypnotic phenomena and an effort to maintain them. Therefore, with appropriate hypnotic treatment planning, these unconscious facets of resistance can be accessed and utilized as a treatment strategy rather than becoming a deterrent to change. So we encourage you not to avoid or challenge resistance but to respect and embrace your client's innocent defenses.

As a hypnotherapist, you will encounter two types or layers of resistance. The first, which the novice likely fears the most, simply involves the client actively or passively resisting the use or induction of hypnosis. The second, which all therapists encounter, is the client's preference for the safety of maladaptive behavior over the uncertainty and anxiety of change. For the purposes of treatment planning we are suggesting that they are one and the same. Many clients who have fears of losing control are also likely to be apprehensive about using hypnosis. They might regard it as mind control or expect that they will feel or say something unexpected.

Obviously, an explanation about the safety of hypnosis will probably not allay a client's adaptive resistance. Nonetheless, it is important to provide a rudimentary education about hypnosis. By taking the time to prepare your client, you will have an opportunity to assess the depth and nature of a client's resistance. Using the everyday examples we have highlighted previously can be a good starting point. You might describe an example of trance as a naturally occurring phenomenon, such as the moment when they are first awakening in the morning, feeling very relaxed under their comfortable covers. Should the client respond, "That never happens to me! I always wake up and bound right out of bed!", you can be fairly certain you are encountering significant resistance. In such a situation, you can continue to explain trance whereby the focus involves control rather than relaxation. You might ask the client if she is the kind of person who can think so deeply about something that she can shut out the rest of the world. By providing an example of hypnotic phenomena, in this case a voluntary dissociation, she will likely find the idea of hypnosis to be less threatening.

The assessment of your client's level of resistance will also be valuable in determining which hypnotic interventions could be most useful, as well as fundamental in determining how change in therapy will likely occur. The treatment plan as a whole will need to incorporate interventions that the client experiences as volitional, if not intentional. As we indicated in the previous chapter, the use of permissive language is preferable when attempting to disrupt a client's conscious and usually rigid perceptions. Being able to choose among alternatives rather than having to accept or reject a single direct suggestion puts the client in charge of his experience. Likewise, clients typically feel frustrated by whatever dilemma they are facing. The modeling of choice through permissive language can instill cooperation and hope. A typical example of this is a technique referred to as "covering all possibilities" (Yapko, 1995). For example, you might predict, "Perhaps you will enter trance quickly, or perhaps more slowly, or in some other way which feels most natural to you." In essence, you provide a number of alternatives that make it difficult not to respond in the direction you are suggesting.

Two very powerful techniques in disrupting rigid thought processes are *reframing* (Bandler & Grinder, 1979; Watzlawick et al., 1974) and the use of *presuppositions* (Haley, 1973). Reframing is essentially the interpretation of a problem by identifying its positive aspects. What could be positive about chronic pain or a significant loss? Often the success of reframing lies in being able to zero in on parts of the whole and finding in those parts something that is positive or productive. Thus, with the chronic pain client, pain can be reframed as the body's signaling system, alerting the client to a physical ailment. However, this signal might be set at a volume that is greater or more constant than the person needs. In this case, hypnosis could be used in toning down the signal to a more manageable level. While this method occasionally feels like you're performing mental gymnastics, you will have changed the client's meaning of symptoms to paradoxically offer a win-win solution. The choice will be to continue her tight grasp on what has been reframed as a positive symptom or to choose another path altogether.

Don't be surprised if a client spontaneously slips into a mini-trance when you have successfully reframed a negative into a positive. It is exciting to see a client shaken out of his fixed frame of reference and, with eyes wide open and mouth agape, say, "I never thought of it like that." Reframing tends to neutralize the noxious aspects of a symptom while also helping the client to identify and address facets of their dilemma that previously seemed unmanageable. Perhaps another way to say this is that a good reframe will turn their view of the symptom upside down. It will never be perceived quite the same way again.

One of my (MD) earliest introductions to reframing came in the first few lines of *Families and Family Therapy*, by Salvador Minuchin (1974), in which he describes the initial moments of an inpatient family therapy session:

Minuchin: What is the problem?
Mr. Smith: I think it's my problem.
Minuchin: Don't be so sure. Never be so sure.
Mr. Smith: Well...I'm the one in the hospital and everything.
Minuchin: Yeah, still that doesn't tell me it is your problem.

Rather than answering Minuchin's query about *what* the problem is, Mr. Smith presents *himself* as the problem. His self-image as an incompetent, ineffectual man becomes immediately evident. This is a man who, after three hospitalizations, is in danger of becoming a professional patient. Minuchin bypasses the particulars of his circumstances and instead challenges Mr. Smith's habituated frame of reference, suggesting that he may have the wrong idea about himself and his situation.

Reframing can be especially useful with resistant clients who fear losing control during hypnosis. They are, as we identified earlier, the ones who will deny ever having the common types of everyday trance. By reframing their need for control and seeding positive, control-taking presuppositions, you can establish a groundwork for successful and collaborative trance work. The presupposition is a form of indirect suggestion that speaks simultaneously to the conscious and unconscious. The conscious mind is directed to curious details such as when, how, or where the change will occur, while the unconscious hears the embedded suggestion that a change is going to happen. For example, you might say, *"You are in such control* of your experience (reframe of resistance) that *hypnosis will be perfect for you* (suggestion). *You decide* (reframe of resistance) just *how comfortable you can become* (presupposition) during the experience. And you won't *allow yourself* (reframe of resistance) to go into trance too quickly" (presupposition).

Although we are highlighting the use of reframing and presupposition with resistant clients, these are interventions that should be used generously with all clients. People usually engage in therapy because they are suffering from a kind of tunnel vision. Like a horse wearing blinders, they may be able to trudge through their daily existence, but they are missing a lot of the scenery and many potential alternative routes. Reframing and presupposition are gentle, effective ways to remove the blinders and let the client see more possibilities.

Mary Anne believed that nothing in her life ever turned out well. In addition to difficulties at work and her apparent inability to develop a long-lasting romantic attachment, she was now facing the prospect of a second face-lift. Her first surgery had been unsuccessful if not traumatic, and she was panicked about going through this excruciatingly painful procedure again. She appeared depressed, with a frozen, flat affect and vocal tone. Her facial expressions were equally unresponsive, except for an occasional smile that seemed ingenuine and forced. I (MD) found rapport-building with her to be laborious, as it took several sessions for me adjust to her inanimate and detached presentation.

During her childhood, Mary Anne was given responsibilities well beyond her years and capacities. She entered adulthood expecting life to be full of burdens that she might not be able to manage. Her response was to feel victimized and fearful of being overwhelmed and immobilized. She was constantly bracing herself physically and emotionally as a way to prepare for the next disappointment. Thus, even when she would risk happiness, she would remain tense and guarded.

To make matters more challenging, she believed that she could not be hypnotized. Why should that be possible when nothing else worked for her?

Rather than attempting to reassure her that she could, I suggested that she had particular talents that would assist us in using hypnosis, even though (of course) we could not be certain that it would work. I asked if she had ever become so worried about something that she lost track of what she was doing. Knowing this to be a typical occurrence of waking-state dissociation, I could predict that she would confirm that this happened all the time. Taking this reframe one step further, I added that not everyone could concentrate so exquisitely. In fact, I told her, this talent for focused concentration is one of the hallmarks of a good hypnotic subject.

My hypnotic induction would need to demonstrate for Mary Anne that she was fully in control and that her unconscious could make its own choices. Having already reframed her rigid negativity as a hypnotic talent, I also wanted to accentuate these abilities through my induction language. Therefore, I decided to use the eye fixation technique that could both validate her control and utilize her adaptive resistance. In order to deepen her trance and not disrupt the experience, I wanted to engage her tendency to obsess. Thus, I suggested that she would find herself questioning some of my statements and that some of these questions might seem more important than the things I was saying to her. I reassured her that as she went into trance (presupposition), she could *go on thinking* about those questions. I also indicated that, because her ability to concentrate was so well developed (reframe), her ability to concentrate would automatically focus (presupposition) on anything that would be helpful for her.

By "going with the resistance," Mary Anne was able to achieve a very enjoyable trance, and much of her future resistance would be diminished. Upon reorienting, she said, "Wow! I never thought it would work! Was I really hypnotized?" I asked if she had followed the directive about critiquing my suggestions and she replied, "Of course. Well, I think I did, at least for a while."

Mary Anne called me following her face-lift procedure. She was giggling as she related how during surgery her surgeon repeatedly asked her if she was okay. While no amount of Valium seemed to quell her anxiety throughout the first procedure, this time she had remained calm, to the surprise and concern of her surgeon.

By utilizing and transforming resistance into a successful validation of hypnotic talent, you can assist your clients in two ways. First, they learn that, despite their doubts and apprehensions, they are hypnotizable. Second, they will have a trance-ratifying experience that will be ego-enhancing and reassuring for both therapist and client. Erickson (Erickson et al., 1976) was often quoted as saying, "How do you know what you know that you didn't know you know?" The self-discovery made possible through hypnosis can build a powerful impetus for future change.

It has been reported that Erickson would hypnotize clients and project them into the future to a time after their treatment had been successfully completed (Erickson, 1954). The client would tell him what kinds of things Erickson had done to help bring about the changes. Erickson then used this information as the basis for his treatment plan. Once you have gained some credibility with the resistant client and through a successful trance experience, you might want to use a variation of this technique. For example, during trance, your client could encounter her wiser, more experienced 80-year-old self who can provide valuable foresight and guidance. The advantages of this intervention are threefold. First, it is the client, not you, who advises herself about what she can do to change. Secondly, it presupposes that the client has progressed in life to a stage of wisdom. In both ways, you are instilling hope and providing ego enhancement. Lastly, such projections into the future can reveal helpful information toward achieving a valid, egosyntonic direction for change.

HYPNOTIC METAPHORS AND BYPASSING CONSCIOUS RESISTANCE

The use of stories and metaphors to teach and heal is as old as civilization (Campbell, 1949). Their effectiveness is rooted in their capacity to bypass conscious or logical examination while addressing the person's concerns on an unconscious level. One does not have to rely on classic literature to find metaphors. The can be found in popular culture, humor, music, and personal or clinical anecdotes. They can be read from books, quoted from memory, or simply made up. Originality and imitation are equally effective.

Early in my training, I (MD) was confused by the use of metaphor in hypnosis. Based on my experience to that point, I believed that I would need to spontaneously construct elaborate, suggestion-laden stories with profound clinical results. My anxiety intensified after I studied for several days with Milton Erickson. Although he was bound to a wheelchair, soft-spoken, and mostly paralyzed on one side, Erickson's stories were captivating. Approximately one hour into the first day's session, I became fatigued and sleepy. I shifted around, doodled, and yawned, but continued to lose ground. Eventually, I realized, "You dummy, this is what you are supposed to do: go into trance." And so I did. Erickson had been seeding suggestions all along toward this outcome. The ease with which he could coax his students and clients into trance, simply by telling stories, left me in awe. Thus, I continued to fret over whether I would ever be able to create a story with such eloquence and subtlety.

I was trying too hard.

Ironically, what helped the most was the 1988 PBS series *Joseph Campbell and the Power of Myth* (1988), in which Bill Moyers interviewed this expert on the myths and cultures of the world. Campbell's enthusiasm for the subject matter was infectious. He told story after story, ranging from the cultures of ancient Greece and India, to the Native Americans, to our modern-day legends such as *Star Wars* (1977). He cited these many, diverse examples to illustrate how people use stories to make sense of their world. He described how people cannot logically explain the mysteries of life, and thus resort to metaphor, stories or poetry as a means to make sense of that which seems inexplicable. It was especially fascinating to hear how Campbell found instances of stories from so many varied cultures and eras that illustrate the human dilemma regarding choice. As he puts it, there are two basic choices in life: "the right-handed path," which is the practical, logic-driven path, or the "left-handed path," which is the riskier path. The latter is also what Campbell calls "following your bliss," because taking this path results in its own rewards.

Our myths are filled with stories of those who take the "left-handed path," or embark on what has also been labeled "the hero's journey." The hero, whether Luke Skywalker of *Star Wars*, Pocahontas, or Gandhi, is usually a common person who finds himself thrust into a strange world. Not only must heroes find a way to survive, but also they are likewise challenged to triumph over incredible odds. Like Arthur with the sword in the stone, they have no idea that a life-changing journey is about to ensue.

It is not difficult to grasp how these themes apply to psychotherapy. Usually something critical has occurred that results in the client seeking therapy. Perhaps she has lost her job or husband. Maybe he is someone with a serious illness, or who feels like a failure as a parent, or who struggles with his excesses of tobacco, alcohol, or food. Possibly, it is simply someone who has taken the "right-handed path" and is idled by ennui or depression. He knows something has to change, yet may not realize that it is he who must change.

Whether the threat is internal or external, our clients must take action and may feel frightened or confused regarding how to address and overcome their present dilemmas. To be successful, they may have to break some rules or taboos to succeed. Or like the hero, they may need to think and act "outside the box" and begin down the left-handed path. That is, their normal way of operating based upon socialization and a defensive structure that is outmoded needs fine-tuning if not a major overhaul. In short, they must become the hero of their own story. This is a fanciful way to describe the work of therapy, and the essential role that the client plays in her own recovery.

The reason we like stories is because they speak to our unconscious. They are universal. When we hear a story, the dilemma does not seem to be about us, it is about someone else. Thus, we can relax and listen. In other words, a story allows us to think we are a passive listener, not someone to whom a message is being given. We are entertained, while the potential lessons of the story seep into and begin percolating in our unconscious.

Stories need not be elaborate. Performance anxiety about needing to be Hemingway or Erickson impedes the natural creativity that can emerge between the client and therapist during the therapy session. To the contrary, a therapeutic metaphor can be an anecdote about something rather trivial that conveys a point. My (MD) clients have become accustomed to my asking, "Did I tell you the story about…?" For example, one of my favorite anecdotes is about the time my mother experienced an infection in the nail bed of her finger when I was a child. I explain to the client that no amount of home remedies or medical intervention was having a lasting effect. Then, one day, while washing dishes, a chip of glass emerged from the infected wound. My mother had forgotten about breaking a drinking glass a few weeks previously. A piece of it had become lodged in her finger, causing the problem. The story usually ends with something along the lines of,

"It wasn't until that painful item was released that the finger became whole again."

I (RV), on the other hand, will often use song lyrics or humorous one-liners to make my point. I make references to other clients' stories as well. These examples might sometimes be disguised personal chapters of my own life. When the subject matter isn't too revealing (or embarrassing) I might even disclose situations I have confronted and managed successfully or unsuccessfully. Annie, an 11-year-old girl, reacted negatively to my suggestion that her mother needed to begin applying logical consequences to control her behavior. I told Annie about how I had trained my dog Shamus (always present in my office) to be such a good pet. I told her how he was crate-trained first so that he would learn to "hold it" until he could be allowed to go outside for important business. When I could trust him, he graduated to an indoor fence. As he increasingly learned to manage the freedom without destroying his bedding or toys, I enlarged his space. When his behavior regressed and he demonstrated an inability to handle this much freedom, I would make the space smaller. Every time he showed me I could trust him, he was given more room. Each week following the story, Annie would ask me if Shamus had been good and was his "room" getting bigger. She ceased her resistance to her mother's efforts and began working hard to earn the trust she deserved.

The Roots and Construction of Metaphor

As we have said, metaphor takes many forms. Yes, it can be a fairy tale or legend that carries great profundity and impact. It can also be a lyric, a joke, or an anecdote. We believe that one of the primary reasons people are drawn to certain movies, music, or books is that the message behind their stories' surface qualities carries a special meaning to the one who is reacting. Even melodies and photographs carry themes that can evoke tears or excitement.

There are two essential ingredients to the spontaneous development of a metaphor. First and obviously, you must understand the unspoken meanings and existential subtext of your client's needs. You will want these "informal" stories to match your client's symptom formation and to offer new alternatives. Remember that it is the goal of metaphor to help your client see her difficulties and potential solutions with "new eyes." Second, you need to have access to and to utilize your own associations. Beyond having a sufficient grasp of your client's needs, there is really little potential harm in going with your instincts. If you are sitting with your client, free associating to what you are seeing and hearing, and you discover that you are simultaneously thinking of something else, chances are you have a metaphor in the making. You will simply put this association into a form that is appropriate and understandable to your listener. I did not plan to talk about Shamus's training; it just occurred to me.

We were recently watching an interview with Julianne Moore on an episode of *Inside the Actor's Studio* (2002). Those of you who are familiar with this program know that the interviews are in-depth and candid. Ms. Moore impressed both of us by saying that the hardest thing for her to learn about acting was to trust herself. She said that for years she couldn't fathom what her professors meant by this. Now that she does, she has provided some of the best screen portrayals of complicated women seen in recent times. Like seeds in a garden, you cannot force your creativity or your unconscious resources to blossom, but you can create the optimal conditions for this to happen. This means being in the moment and paying attention to what is present in the interaction, not focusing upon doing it well.

I (MD) treated Alice intermittently for several years. Her emotional development was admirable and I felt honored to work with her. During one recent spring, we were working together only sporadically. Although she was only 52 years old, the effects of chemotherapy treatments 25 years earlier were finally catching up with her. A few months into this episode of treatment, she learned that her condition was fatal. In the time we had left, Alice prepared herself and her loved ones for her death.

Our last few sessions were held in her home. As I drove to what turned out to be our last session, I was filled with dread. I knew that Alice was looking to me for help in facing death and had requested that we use hypnosis to ease her fears about dying. Having lost my father just months earlier to a very similar set of symptoms, I was afraid that my grief for them both would overwhelm me and I would disappoint Alice when she needed me most. Walking to her door, I was reminding myself, "This is about Alice, not you."

My fears were groundless, in the sense that Alice provided us with the material we needed. She said she knew it was time for her to go. Not only had her condition worsened considerably, but also she had received a "message" from her grandmother. Being Jewish, Alice had lit the Sabbath candle the evening before. It was their custom to leave the candles burning in a safe place even after they went to bed. During her sleep, Alice dreamed of her grandmother, who said, "Your time for lighting candles is over." Alice believed her grandmother was waiting for her, but she feared her family and friends were not ready for her to go. What could she do to help both them and herself deal with this separation?

As Alice drifted in and out of trance, I was able to relate various things I had learned about this very issue during my father's illness and death. Like my father, Alice had difficulty accepting help. I knew that, as her condition worsened, she would become more and more debilitated. My father, always the caretaker, had graciously accepted our help with even the most basic of functions. It was an honor to be able to give my father the kind of nursing he needed. Alice was surprised that this was one of the things that made my father's death more acceptable to me. I told her that it helped me to feel as though I had done what I could to make his passage better. We couldn't stop his illness or the fact that he was leaving, but we could make it the best farewell possible. Alice died two weeks later.

During that last visit, Alice, knowing of my strong Irish heritage, gave me a pin she had bought in Ireland. The pin was a small painting of the site of King Cormac's Chapel. Alice did not know that my father's name is Cormac.

Although creating metaphors might seem like 99 percent inspiration, there are a few guidelines that will help in making them effective. The more you immerse yourself in stories, the easier it will become to let your own emerge. Again, whatever your particular areas of interest are, whether they are sports, gardening, skydiving, cooking, or crafts, these can be the basis of your stories. The story is the message; the content is the window dressing.

Joseph Campbell assisted George Lucas in creating the story lines for the initial *Star Wars* trilogy. Luke Skywalker's development is a wonderful example of the hero's journey. The following are key elements (adapted from Campbell & Moyers, 1988; and Pearson, 1991) in creating an effective therapeutic tale, with Luke's story as our model.

1. *Theme*. Theme should correspond to the client's particular dilemma in order to be effective. Thus, imagining your client as the main character of your football, gardening, or culinary tale, you can introduce conflicts which mirror your client's problem or the challenges she is facing. Luke, a typical teenager, is restless. He has developed certain skills, such as executing daring aeronautical feats in his speeder, but feels stuck and constrained by his circumstances. He wants adventure, but

feels an obligation to his family. A crisis occurs in which his family is destroyed, and he sets off to avenge them and learn about the "Force."

2. *Helpers*. Every hero sometimes needs help. Thus, helpers in the form of actual people bearing the client's attributes or unconscious resources need to be represented. Even if your hero must face a challenge alone, the helpers prepare her for this journey into the unknown. Obi-Wan, R2D2, C3PO, and Hans Solo are Luke's initial helpers. They reflect different aspects of a whole person. Some of these are: wisdom (Obi-Wan), technical ability (R2D2), book learning and caution (C3PO), and humor and street smarts (Han Solo). When Princess Leia joins them, she becomes the doorway to the new world.

3. *Challenge. and success*. The hero will be challenged, perhaps by what may seem to be unbeatable odds. However, through her own wits and with the help given by her assistants, she succeeds. Luke must enter the belly of the beast and rescue the princess. He incorporates the wisdom of his teacher who has perished. With his helpers and his own unconscious resources, Luke not only rescues the princess, but also destroys the evil that threatens their world.

4. *New identity*. By facing the challenge, the hero stretches beyond his known capacities. He discovers resources and strengths he doesn't know he has. His view of himself must likewise expand, as he no longer resides in his old world. He has entered a new dimension. Luke is no longer a boy. Trusting his instincts, he has succeeded where others have failed. He is becoming a man.

5. *Wholeness and affirmation*. The hero overcomes fear and thus has become better integrated as a whole self. This wholeness is acknowledged and celebrated by herself, and often her entire community. In the final scene, the entire community of the New Republic gathers to honor Luke and his friends. He is acknowledged as having faced down the demons that threatened his world.

Although structuring therapeutic tales may seem daunting, as Obi-Wan advises, "Use the Force, Luke," or in other words, give your unconscious free rein. The pieces will fall into place. A story, however, is only as good as its reception. As you use metaphor with your clients, you will be able to tell if you are hitting the mark by their nonverbal responses. If you are telling a metaphor with a client who is not in a formal trance, you will likely see the telltale signs of nonverbal agreement, such as head nods, slowed breathing, or rapt eye contact. If a client is in trance, you may see some of the same nonverbal behaviors, or it may appear as though she is going further into trance. In other words, be certain you are remaining in rapport with your client as you use metaphor.

Regardless of the source of your inspirations, we urge you to follow them. As long as the message of your story or reference is hopeful and true, there is little chance of causing harm and a reasonable probability of doing a great deal of good. After hearing a metaphor, it is not uncommon for a client to remark, "Yes, that reminds me of when...," which is a rather sure sign you have engaged her unconscious in the story's meaning.

On occasion, your client will let you know where you have gone wrong. Early in my (RV) hypnotic work with Carla, she described her "safe place" as the bank of a stream where she would sit on the grass and look across to the lush greenery on the other side. The stream was shallow enough that rocks showed through all the way to the other side. The presence of these rocks intrigued me, and I thought perhaps they were there for a purpose. In a subsequent hypnosis session, I suggested she could stand and begin walking, from one rock to the next, to the other side. A troubled expression fell over her face, and I asked if she would like to tell me what was happening. The current of the stream had increased to the point where rapids now covered the rocks. She could not cross.

Since every detail of her fantasy was a projection of herself, there was a new message here, a new part of her being revealed. Carla was telling me that she was not prepared to cross the stream. In retrospect, this was the first indication of her dissociative disorder. Carla wanted to cross, but some other part of her did not. We now use this metaphor as a kind of goal. One day all the parts of her will be ready to see and feel the other side, together.

On occasion, a metaphor will be handed right to you. Jeremy was referred to me (RV) by his pediatrician for trichotillomania, an anxiety disorder that features the absentminded pulling of hair. The source of Jeremy's anxiety was primarily his military father, who was equally authoritarian in his work and family life. His verbal abuse and threatening behavior made everyone tense, particularly his children. During one session with 10-year-old Jeremy, his mother related something he had said to her after our last session. He had told her that he felt that he was at a "Y in the road." His choice was to either take the "rickety bridge" of confronting his father or to go "back into the swamp" of accepting orders and tolerating abuse. This is an amazingly mature boy whose poise and insight are well beyond his years. With the assistance of his imagination, we have our beginning point for hypnosis and the possibility of a number of metaphors. Jeremy's disclosure indicates that a major focus will be upon ego strengthening to help him choose which course he truly wishes to follow.

IDEOMOTOR SIGNALING: CONVERSATIONS WITH THE UNCONSCIOUS MIND

Our primary assumptions in using hypnosis are that the unconscious is a powerful influence in every aspect of a client's functioning and that we wish to make contact with these potentials for some therapeutic gain. From the deepest levels of body management, memory retention, and repression, much of the action is beneath conscious awareness. As with other hypnotic phenomena, ideomotor behavior is the natural expression of unconscious process via observable physiological behavior (blushing, head nods, etc.) (Yapko, 2003). In treatment, we learn to read and interpret these expressions as a means of understanding a client's underlying genuine needs and emotions. We also initiate communication with a client's unconscious by suggesting a means of "speaking" through specifically identified involuntary messages. With the use of finger signaling, pendulums, and other methods, we gently and carefully "question" the unconscious without contaminating its content with new information.

Although Erickson is credited as the first to develop ideomotor signaling, he limited its use ostensibly to induction and deepening and as a trance-ratifying technique (Weitzenhoffer, 1989). It has since gained great popularity for unconscious exploration and reintegration, thanks to the contributions of David Cheek, Cory Hammond, and others (Rossi & Cheek, 1988; Hammond & Cheek, 1988). Our coverage of these techniques is intended to be brief, while highlighting how it can be a particularly effective tool in bypassing resistance. We recommend further reading by the above authors and/or attending a workshop in which its use is demonstrated and practiced by participants.

Humans have a tendency to behave in self-defeating ways. They say that they want one thing only to have their wishes undermined by uncooperative and contrary unconscious motivations. Such is the nature of resistance. In these cases, we might investigate the sources of these contradictions and bypass conscious resistance by seeking the assistance of the unconscious more directly. While the use of metaphors can similarly serve this function, ideomotor signaling involves a more active and immediate client-therapist interaction.

Probably the most common method of ideomotor signaling is the technique where the client's unconscious is asked to assign different fingers with which it might answer questions. First, it is suggested to the hypnotized client that he repeatedly think of the word "yes." The therapist requests that the unconscious choose a finger to lift on their nondominant hand to signify the "yes" response. This procedure is followed with the answers "No," and also, "I don't know/I don't want to answer." If the client is anxious or impatient, he may try to "help" by consciously lifting his finger. This rapid or forceful movement indulges its conscious origins while impeding a more authentic unconscious response. Should this be the case, you might respectfully acknowledge the willful participation of the conscious mind and then again suggest that the unconscious take its time in "allowing" the correct finger to gently rise. You will usually recognize unconscious finger responses as characterized by their subtle, sometimes imperceptible movements. Should the answer be difficult to discern, you might simply suggest that the responding finger will gently lift a bit more in making its intentions more apparent.

While finger signaling is probably the most straightforward means of ideomotor communication, the attachment of behaviors to unconscious answers can take many forms. The hypnotherapist can be creative in utilizing the client's idiosyncratic ideomotor movements by assigning a meaning to those movements. I (MD) was first introduced to ideomotor signaling as a demonstration subject with Dr. Cheek. My request was that he help me to manage a certain physical discomfort I was experiencing. Noticing that I had been fidgeting with my ring, he offered the post-hypnotic suggestion that, whenever my pain returned, that my unconscious would automatically remind me to twist the ring to "turn around the pain."

The choice of a signal can also originate from your client's spontaneous ideomotor behavior. For example, Julie (MD) suffered chronic depression partially resulting from a dissociation from her egodystonic feelings of anger and frustration. She was irrationally fearful of offending others and avoided confrontation whenever possible, thus requiring that she acquiesce to demands and repress her true wishes. While exploring these issues in trance, I asked her unconscious to signal whenever she was uncomfortable with any of my requests.

Several minutes passed before her nose began twitching. She broke into a huge smile, saying, "Gosh, my nose is itching! It is really itching!" After she made this connection, Julie's nose would itch whenever her unconscious wished to say, "No."

Ideomotor signaling can be used in a number of ways during hypnosis. For example, you could instruct the client to signal with a "yes" response when they have reached a comfortable level of trance, when they have completed a piece of hypnotic work such as an unconscious dream, or when they are ready for the next suggestion. These applications merely provide the client and her unconscious with a convenient, unobtrusive means of communicating.

For our purposes, we wish to emphasize that ideomotor signaling allows us to decipher the bases for enigmatic barriers to progress. Since resistance is an unconscious effort to protect oneself, it is essential to respect this misguided intent even as you seek to therapeutically alter its expression. Through the use of ideomotor signaling, we are allowed to investigate the need for self-protection without actually challenging it. Once we gain new insights regarding the resistant behavior, we can more accurately pursue alternative solutions. Should these barriers involve overwhelming, emotionally laden memories, we then use signaling to help us to pace our interventions and monitor unconscious readiness through direct feedback from the unconscious.

For the apprehensive hypnotherapist, ideomotor signaling offers solutions for many of the more difficult situations he will face. It allows him to delicately proceed with the potentially fragile or volatile trauma victim. It offers a method through which confounding, counterproductive behaviors might be understood. The greatest dread for any psychotherapist is failure, yet failure in treatment often represents success for unconscious needs and motivations. Ideomotor signaling can lead to explanations and alternatives for adaptive resistance.

CHAPTER 7

Treatment Planning:
Basic Steps

In the process of writing this book, we find ourselves in somewhat of a bind. It is customary with a work of this length to break a subject down into chapters that each covers some key element of its message. We have made an effort to do just that. However, we do not want to perpetuate or promote the misconception that hypnosis is a sequence of unrelated stages or techniques, one after the other. We don't necessarily even want to suggest that hypnosis begins with the induction and ends in reorientation.

In essence, we hope that, as you integrate hypnosis into your practice, you will begin to *think hypnotically* throughout your work and with all clients. We have aspired to make clear how a client expresses hypnotic phenomena through their symptoms; how these phenomena can be used as the doorway to trance induction; and finally, how the alteration and/or expansion of these phenomena through hypnosis can lead to lasting changes. As you begin to grasp the role of natural trance and hypnotic language throughout treatment, your comfort with the process will accelerate. In the process, the client learns that she has a wealth of strengths and resources, some of which she has long considered to be liabilities.

Thus, when we speak of the hypnotic relationship, we are not just describing the period of time in which the therapist and client use formal trance. Ideally, hypnosis begins when a therapist first talks with a prospective client, and, ideally, it doesn't end at all. From first contact, a hypnotherapist is learning about his client, providing reassurance and information, and establishing the groundwork for a hypnotic relationship. We would hope and expect that, when treatment has ended, the client will have learned how to access and use the powers of her own unconscious more deliberately and more constructively.

So, instead of viewing hypnosis in stages, which suggests a linear process, we suggest that hypnosis occurs in *layers*. Thus each layer is separate in and of itself and simultaneously fused with, and influenced by, the other layers. The therapist seizes upon the unique talents of an individual in conducting a hypnotic session that is both reflective of and complementary to those talents. The client's hypnotic strengths will become the focal point with the introduction of treatment and will be utilized for trance induction and treatment, and their expression and composition will possibly be altered in a constructive way.

Figure 7.1 is a graphic representation of how this might look:

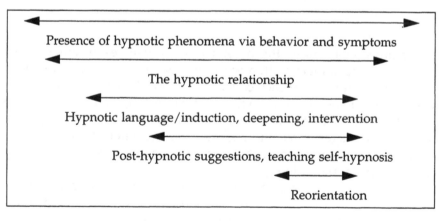

Figure 7.1

This diagram highlights the fact that the client enters and leaves her encounter with you demonstrating preexisting hypnotic talents. Although these talents have previously served to both protect and inhibit her growth, the client may conclude therapy with these same talents intact, but altered and redirected toward growth. The hypnotic relationship and the therapist's use of hypnotic language begin prior to the induction and continue throughout treatment. The induction, deepening, and further application of trance merely build upon this relationship for the duration of the hypnotic session.

Barbara, a third-year medical student, was referred by her physician for pain management. Over the past year, cramping during her menstrual cycle had resulted in her missing much of her school year. Medical tests had revealed no pathological process to explain the severity of her discomfort. She was now on probation and feared she would be expelled if her grades didn't soon improve. Although she had been prescribed pain relievers, these did little to relieve her suffering. In fact, Barbara entered my (MD) office slightly bent, holding her abdomen and looking several years older than her age of 24. During our first interview, she winced in pain and fidgeted in her chair, trying to find a comfortable way to sit.

Barbara was angry at her pain, complaining, "It's destroying my life!" Aware that we were only just beginning to know and understand each other, I cautiously suggested, "I would bet that your pain is doing quite the contrary." At first Barbara seemed dumbstruck (another term for momentary trance), and said angrily, "You think I want this pain? Do you think I am making this up?" I replied, "No, of course not. I just think your body is trying to tell you something. We just don't understand yet what the message is."

Barbara's history revealed that she had grown up in a fairly perfectionist family where only her retarded younger sister was excused from being exceptional. She had not only graduated from college with a double major after only three and a half years, but she had also been admitted to a prestigious medical school. Even so, the disruption this pain was causing in her life made her both furious and defeated.

In following the "layers of hypnosis" paradigm suggested earlier, we begin by viewing Barbara in terms that would be helpful in treatment planning. It is obvious that Barbara entered treatment demonstrating a number of hypnotic talents and that, since she arrived at sessions in obvious pain, avoiding that fact or trying to minimize it would only create strain and resistance, not a sense of ease. The hypnotic relationship is facilitated by reflecting back to the client the very hypnotic phenomena that may be supporting her symptoms. Their inclusion in the induction communicates to the client and her unconscious an empathic connection that goes beyond words. Therefore, these talents were utilized with Barbara as the basis for appropriate hypnotic language as well as in achieving induction and deepening.

To begin with, Barbara was emotionally cataleptic, feeling frustrated by her inability to move out of her present pattern of pain and frustration. She was paralyzed by conflicts and solutions from childhood (age regression), limiting her choices and expectations of herself. Hypersthesia was evident both emotionally and physically through her hypersensitivity to perceived criticism and preoccupation with physical pain. Likewise, when she was in pain, time seemed endless, thus time distortion was evident as well. Barbara's sensory strengths would be a consideration as well. As her symptoms suggested, she was highly kinesthetic, so our language and imagery would respect and incorporate such a preference.

I was able to establish accurate empathy by recognizing and joining with Barbara's motivation to feel physically better and more competent. I did this by reframing her symptom into a communication from her body, not a senseless saboteur of her life plans. I redirected her physical hypervigilance to identify areas of her body that experienced either less discomfort or actual comfort.

As the layered model suggests, my induction was but a continuation of this language. Barbara was asked to focus upon her discomfort and, in particular, to notice its various means of expression. For example, at different times, it might feel like a stabbing sensation, a dull wave of discomfort, or she might even notice a particular warmth in the discomfort. To reflect the time expansion and the cognitive distortions of age regression, I suggested that "As you notice the various ways in which the discomfort expresses itself, you may also wonder when it will end? How soon can you feel better again?" It might be helpful to remind the reader that one does not have to be relaxed or even comfortable to enter trance. Barbara provides a good example of someone whose focused absorption lies in her pain and frustration. We utilized this focus and her hypnotic talents to induce trance and to achieve a greater breadth of trance.

Finally, intervention consisted of utilizing her physical pain as a starting point for reaching back to its origin and purpose. While she was in trance, I (MD) suggested that Barbara could go back to the period in her life when her symptoms first began. Barbara was surprised to recall an incident when, at the age of 13, her parents excused her from attending a church function. Still in trance, Barbara began laughing. "I hated those damn socials!" she exclaimed. "I guess I figured out how to get out of that one." It was suggested that her unconscious mind could find other ways in which to allow her "a way out" when she needed a break. With the suggestion that time was speeding up and she was now in the midst of her next menstrual cycle, Barbara was asked to see how her unconscious had helped her resolve the problem. She visualized soaking in a hot bath, reading a "steamy novel." When asked if this would be an acceptable substitute for the pain, Barbara exclaimed, "Damn straight!" It was then suggested that she imagine a time when menstrual pain might somehow come in handy. She smiled and nodded her head; "When my folks want me to come home from school for a weekend to relax. If I want to relax, I want to do it with my friends!" Suggestions were made for having just enough pain, for just long enough, to allow Barbara to feel entitled to refusing her parents' invitation.

Barbara's unconscious, by incapacitating her physically, had created an appropriate "solution" to the demands she placed upon herself. Although this had been an acceptable solution when she was 13, at 24 it was debilitating to her and evoked feelings of incompetence. Hypnosis allowed her to develop alternatives that went beyond work at the office. Like the first domino tumbling, Barbara's letting go of the pain helped her develop a number of ways in which to "get away" from responsibility without feeling guilty. These solutions became the basis of the post-hypnotic suggestions, which also included the idea that Barbara would naturally find herself learning more about her needs and wishes. Perhaps one of those discoveries led Barbara to taking more time for herself generally.

It is noteworthy that Barbara's new solution, hot baths and "steamy novels," reflected her sensory preferences while addressing what was lacking in her life. The problem for which she sought treatment was tactilely based and she was overworking her mental capacities while being deprived of pleasure. The baths gave her a pleasurable tactile experience to replace the menstrual pain, while also giving her a forum in which to enjoy some intellectual stimulation that was anything but academic!

This layered approach to treatment planning encourages you to first perceive your client in hypnotic terms and then to conceive of a hypnotic "theme" that you will follow throughout therapy. Consider the way in which a composer will adopt a theme and blend its elements throughout the movements of a symphony. Prior to visiting the United States, Czech composer Antonín Dvořák had incorporated the folk music of his Bohemian roots into his classical works. Here he found the melodies of southern slaves to be the most representative of American folk culture. These themes inspired his *New World Symphony,* which maintains the form of a classical composition yet weaves the melodies and motifs of African-American spirituals into the layers of its movements. The fusion of classical form with a rich folk tradition makes the whole truly greater than the sum of its parts. The same is true of the hypnotic relationship, as the therapist practices the form and techniques of hypnosis while embracing the individual client in composing each new "masterpiece."

Just as Dvořák fused classical composition with the African-American melodies to produce a truly original symphony, the alchemy that occurs in the hypnotic relationship provides the basis for a corrective emotional experience. By enlisting and expanding the client's hypnotic talents in the service of her growth, the client, not the therapist, is the composer of these changes. Rossi (1993), in writing about Erickson's novel approach to hypnotic psychotherapy, quotes Erickson as follows:

> The induction and maintenance of a trance serve to provide a special psychological state in which the patient can *re-associate and reorganize his inner psychological complexities and utilize his own capacities in a manner in accord with his own experiential life....* Therapy results from an inner re-synthesis of the patient's behavior *achieved by the patient himself.* It's true that direct suggestion can effect an alteration in the patient's behavior and result in a symptomatic cure, at least temporarily. However, such a "cure" is simply a response to suggestion and does not entail that re-association and reorganization of ideas, understandings and memories so essential for actual cure. It is this experience of re-associating and reorganizing his own experiential life that eventuates in a cure, not the manifestation of responsive behavior which can, at best, satisfy only the observer. (p. 88)

HYPNOTIC TREATMENT PLANNING

For the neophyte hypnotherapist who has learned to induce and deepen trance, treatment planning and intervention are often considered to be most awkward and daunting tasks. Yet it is perhaps the primary purpose of this book to suggest just the opposite. When properly conceived and undertaken, the application of hypnotic skills becomes merely an extension of everything you know to that point. Let us review.

First and most importantly, you are a competent therapist and you are seeing only clientele whom you have been properly trained to treat. Before even considering the use of hypnosis, you will have a general idea of how you would want to proceed with a particular client. Second, you have paid due attention to preparing your client for hypnosis and building rapport. Third, you have identified your client's hypnotic and sensory strengths and have utilized this information in your language. By working from such a foundation built on competence, confidence, and rapport, formal hypnotic work becomes merely a natural extension of the same.

It would be impossible for us to address treatment planning for all clients and diagnostic categories, as the possibilities are essentially infinite. Our intention is not to make such an attempt, but to provide a mindset that can assist you in fusing hypnosis with your existing skills. However, we will discuss what we consider to be three common elements in all hypnotic treatment planning: ego strengthening, the use of imagery, and post-hypnotic suggestion. After a brief discussion of the rare occurrence of unexpected abreactions, we will then apply these principles in treatment planning to two common diagnostic categories: depression and anxiety.

Ego-Strengthening Suggestions

We believe that ego strengthening should be a part of every hypnotherapy session. It is perhaps the most basic and effective means by which to instill hope and prepare the client for change. The initial treatment goal for many of our less-functional clients is stabilization and preparation for more invasive hypnotic interventions. Just as it is often said that psychotherapy is a form of "ego lending," hypnosis can infuse such individuals with empowerment and reaffirmation of dormant strengths. From such a stronger base, alterations and improvements to the client's present functioning can be made more easily.

Nearly everyone who enters psychotherapy suffers from a loss of control in some area of her life. Due to overwhelming or confusing circumstances, some part of her normal, efficient functioning has broken down. Her confidence is limited or absent and hope is nearly lost. Others enter therapy with a historically weak ego functioning, chronically making poor, self-destructive choices and suffering with the results.

Empowerment
Enter hypnosis, which is potentially an empowering experience in itself. Clients are shown their capacity to enter a peaceful, centered

state of consciousness and to experience the awesome capacity of their unconscious to control symptoms, memory, or self-esteem. Additionally, it seems reasonable to include in any hypnotic treatment planning a few post-hypnotic suggestions for improved confidence and strength. We have learned to begin hypnotherapy with positive, trance-ratifying images and to develop a positive mindset or to visit past positive experiences before reconstructive therapy.

We find that with nearly all clients, we include some or all of the following messages within their hypnotic experience:

- Emphasizing the courage they demonstrate in undertaking this new experience.
- Stressing positive anticipation of the relief and constructive changes they will experience.
- Utilizing all experience in hypnosis as natural, normal, and expected.
- Making post-hypnotic suggestions that they will continue to gain confidence, strength, and understanding in a conscious or unconscious way.
- Reinforcing the power of their own unconscious minds to create such calm and deeper understanding.
- Stating all observations and post-hypnotic suggestions in positive terms.

Wonder Is the Beginning of Wisdom

Erickson would routinely speak of his experiences with polio that almost completely immobilized him both as a young man and later in his adult life (Haley, 1973). During his initial illness, he aided his own recovery by observing his younger sister, who was just learning to crawl at the time. He watched with fascination as she used various muscle groups and trial and error to learn how to creep, then crawl, and eventually stand. She was, of course, not conscious of the wondrous learning she was incorporating into her behavioral repertoire, but Erickson was. Not only did he use this knowledge to help himself relearn how to stand and walk, but it also became an integral part of his understanding of human learning and development. He would often incorporate intricate descriptions of an infant's elemental achievements of standing and walking into his inductions with clients. These descriptions not only helped clients access these specific skill sets, but also served to remind them of their natural curiosity and ingenuity that are an integral part of finding the answers they were seeking.

While studying with Erickson, I (MD) experienced this technique firsthand. He spoke of the challenges a baby must face just to be able to elevate herself from a lying position to a crouching or kneeling one. He emphasized how that baby wants to experience something *new*. She does not want to stay passive, observing the same familiar things anymore. The infant does not consider how difficult the task will be, nor does it matter that she doesn't know how to do what she wants to do. Her inquisitiveness is stronger than any caution and her determination overshadows the fact that she is flying blind. While it is often said that Erickson's genius lay in his keen observations, he also effectively exploited these developmental milestones to evoke a desired response. Certainly, if you wish to discover a mother lode of ideas for evoking a client's self-pride and memories of experimentation and success, watch an infant exercising her will in learning to move, stand, and walk. With little effort, ego-enhancing suggestions will begin percolating into your imagination.

Imagery

Hypnoprojective imagery can arise from either of two primary sources. Either we will provide content as a more directive reflection of our client, or he will create his own fantasies as we encourage him through permissive language. Most often, over the course of treatment, we will do both. As we hear the descriptions of his experiences, we will further design images that are increasingly customized.

Anna was a 30-year-old social worker who complained of depression and anxiety attacks. Except for her successes in academic and athletic pursuits, her self-esteem was generally poor and her social life limited. Anna had been both physically and sexually abused by her father. Her dependence on her family for financial and emotional support prevented her from addressing issues with her father and required that she suppress and repress appropriate limits and her reactions to the abuse.

Given her trauma history, I (RV) knew that Anna was understandably gifted in dissociation, anesthesia, and amnesia. Her sensitivity to rejection also suggested talents for positive hallucination and hypermnesia. We undertook psychotherapy and hypnosis to achieve access and management of memory and affect, control over present interpersonal relations, reintegration, and stability.

During the early stages of treatment, our focus was to nurture a mutually trusting, therapeutic relationship sufficient to endure the reconstructive work that would follow. Initial hypnosis was exclusively focused on building a common language, capacity for trance management, and ego strengthening. We also created a setting to which future hypnoprojective work could be added. These images made ample use of her visual and kinesthetic strengths, but I could not foresee the extent to which her talents would take her.

Anna not only created a safe place, a room, but went on to decorate it. She was able to view her childhood on a television screen, beginning at the front door, into her bedroom, and eventually to the abuse that occurred in this room. With only gentle and permissive suggestion, she chose to enter this room and rescue her childhood self, deciding to pummel her father in the process. Her childhood ego state was now a permanent resident of her room, which eventually included her mother and myself.

As Anna began to reconnect with traumatic memories and to reprocess shame into rage, her anger began to overflow and was often displaced in her work and personal relationships. To assist her in managing her anger, we introduced a "safe" where she could store her anger, until it was more manageable.

Later in treatment, Anna carried a familiar theme to a new level of creativity. She decided to attend a weekend trauma survivors' group in a neighboring state. As she was driving to the event, she realized that she would need her anger. She stopped at a rest area off the highway and entered a bathroom stall in the women's room. There she put herself into trance, went to her room, opened her safe, removed her anger, and drove on.

My work with Anna illustrates exactly how imagery can originate from multiple sources. The initial "safe room" image is fairly customary with trauma survivors as a place where other more evocative work might take place. From that point, Anna became a virtual virtuoso in constructing, designing, and creatively utilizing her own fantasy. In fact, I sometimes relate the story of Anna to other clients as a demonstration of the client's retention of control and as a metaphor for the powers of the unconscious in the process of healing.

It is common knowledge that perception is heavily influenced by projection. We see the world through "rose-colored glasses" or "walk around under a dark cloud." All sensory input is filtered through each person's unique fingerprint of conscious and unconscious experience. Our memories, associations, and belief systems color what we hear, see, and feel. We are said to "project" ourselves onto a situation and to make each perception uniquely our own.

Hypnosis utilizes this process by suggesting a projection. Create an opportunity for your client to construct an image — a fantasy, a story, etc. — and you have accessed material unique to that individual. Like a client's responses to Rorschach cards, their interpretation of permissive suggestions is a window into the individual's unconscious processes.

I (MD) recall a projective experience that occurred during a workshop with Erica Fromm. Although Dr. Fromm is typically directive in her approach, on this occasion we were given an indirect suggestion to imagine ourselves someplace special to us. I found myself on the Hawaiian island of Kauai, the gentle breezes blowing and the colors shimmering vibrantly. She suggested that, in whichever way we chose, something in the scene would somehow bring us a message. My mind began to whisper, "Take this peace with you wherever you go." In comparing notes after this experience, one student reported that he was on a mountaintop seeing a message in a cloud. Another found himself by a stream, the crickets' song becoming a signal to go deeper into his trance. Still another found herself in a cross-country marathon in which she could not find the finish line until a volunteer said, "Oh, you passed the finish line long ago." This guided but permissive imagery allowed each of the participants to create whatever projections and suggestions suited us at the time.

We stress the use of your client's interests and sensory strengths whenever possible. This is particularly helpful if you are working with someone who may lack confidence regarding his abilities to either use hypnosis or imagine something on his own. While you are providing much of the content for hypnoprojection, you can be simultaneously permissive by leaving the choice of sensory awareness and many details up to him. A writer or avid reader might be asked to see the pages of a book; a bicyclist might take a smooth, easy ride along a path and observe a scene in the distance; a machinist would understand dials and switches used to increase or decrease pain; a cook can grasp the need to add ingredients sequentially to produce a particular outcome. If you are using the suggestion of a staircase for the purpose of deepening, you might encourage your client to notice how his feet sink into the soft, deep pile of the carpet ("notice the color"), to hear the creaking of the stairs, to see the gleaming wooden banister ("notice what type of wood"), and to smell the roses in a vase on the landing. This "shotgun" approach will likely hit on something that works for the client and ensure a vivid experience for him. The possibilities are endless.

Post-Hypnotic Suggestions: Prompts, Cues, and Attachments

The true measure of successful therapy is what happens outside the clinical setting. Since our purpose is to alter the client's life in some positive way, the client will hopefully begin to think, act, and feel differently than she did prior to treatment. Thus, we need to ask ourselves, "What do I want my client to do after a hypnosis session? Do I want something in particular to happen or not to happen? Do I want the unconscious to provide information we do not yet know? Do I want the client to experience increased affect control to help her manage intense material more safely? Do I want to facilitate greater confidence in my skills and in hypnosis or do I want to stress personal autonomy and ego strengthening?" These are just a few of the factors to consider in choosing a path for post-hypnotic suggestions.

Open and Closed Suggestions

While learning how to perform diagnostic interviews, most clinicians discover the importance of using open- or closed-ended questions and when each approach might be most helpful. Typically, the more we want a client to express himself, the more likely we are to use an open-ended question. When we want a specific bit of information, we will not be so intentionally abstract. Open and closed suggestions are intended to stimulate similar reactions on the client's part.

The more we want the client to create a response from his own repertoire of feelings, ideas, and behaviors, the more likely we are to use open suggestions. An open hypnotic suggestion merely indicates that we do not know (or care) what will happen. We simply want to learn. An open suggestion indicates that we do not know, or have an investment in, how a change will occur. We simply want something to develop which will likely cause the client to learn something new and/or reconnect with something already known, but forgotten. We suggest that the client will gain greater understanding through daydreams, night dreams, or idle thoughts.

Imagine that you are treating a woman who presents with general restlessness, a moderately depressed mood, and yet she reports there are no identifiable difficulties in her life. Although her history suggests competence and resourcefulness, she is now becoming discouraged and losing ground in her work, relationships, and personal growth. Hypnotherapy would initially focus on ego strengthening and accessing internal sources of strength. Yet we want to determine the roots of her rather cryptic symptoms and emotional catalepsy. In this situation, we might use an open suggestion such as, "The unconscious will slowly and safely provide information to the conscious mind that will be helpful in this situation and in a way that will feel comfortable at all times. This information might appear in your dreams or in your idle thoughts, but it will occur in just the right way and at just the right time." By phrasing our suggestions in this way, we are predicting no particular outcome. Furthermore, we have indirectly encouraged our client to become more vigilant to the subtleties of her life that have thus far escaped her attention.

A closed suggestion simply means that we want to limit what will happen in a way that will aid treatment. Because direct or closed post-hypnotic suggestions are risky in that they increase the chances of failure, they should be made only with very compliant, trusting, and motivated clients. For example, your client is seeking help for habit control. Your desired outcome is clear, so there is little room for ambiguity. In such a case, you might suggest, "You will find that your craving is much less frequent and much easier to control." We know what we want to happen, so we suggest it.

Successful Suggestions

Whether they are open or closed, post-hypnotic suggestions should be introduced with as much a chance of success as possible. Obviously, it is your hope that these suggestions will facilitate the relief of symptoms and achievement of the goals that brought your client to treatment. Yet it is perhaps even more important that you build your client's confidence in herself, in the power of her unconscious, in hypnosis, and in the therapist. Just as the language of induction and deepening is built upon presenting hypnotic phenomena and observable behavior, suggestions must be rooted in the inevitable. They must be just vague enough and just specific enough to arouse curiosity. Even if you should suggest no change, you are ensuring that faith in the process will grow. You will later use this faith to promote the outcomes that are truly significant.

With either open or closed suggestions, your familiarity with a client's routines and habits will increase the probability of their realization. Whenever you can approach certainty that events will occur, you increase the chances that both the suggestion and its cue will be perceived as naturally occurring events. The achievement of such a powerful trance ratification and validation of ego strength will contribute greatly toward the success of treatment overall.

Of course, open and indirect suggestions are more likely to be successful than direct or closed ones. The momentum you gain through vague but predictable outcomes can then lead to more pointed and challenging suggestions. For example, you might safely predict that "the unconscious will begin to communicate something that will be helpful in your search...in your thoughts and dreams...and though you might not recognize this at first, when you do, you might not even be aware...that something of importance is beginning to change...but you will know something positive might be about to occur." You can then build upon this limited but recognizable success with, "At some point in the next week...and that might be tomorrow or some other day...a thought will occur to you that will catch your attention...and that thought will stay with you..." In creating post-hypnotic suggestions, success builds upon itself just as your client's resolve will grow with the empowerment of the experience.

We are saying that, at least initially, the success of a suggestion is more valuable than the magnitude of its response. We also wish to emphasize that the language of the suggestion can often predetermine this success. The creative use of words and phrases can evoke the curiosity of the unconscious and set the stage for new insights and the impetus for change.

The direction you take with your creative language will be determined by your treatment goals, your client's hypnotic talents, and the nature of his resistance. For example, when delivering direct suggestions, you might want to increase their likelihood of success by including a bit of deflection. Just as the magician distracts the attention of his audience from his sleight of hand with the flourish of his other hand, you can divert your client's attention from the direct suggestion by adding something that is intellectually captivating. With the above suggestion you might include a phrase such as, "You can be curious about (amazed, surprised, incredulous, etc.) how you find your craving is much less frequent and much easier to control."

Prompts, Cues, and Attachments
Three building blocks to successful suggestions are the inclusion of prompts, cues, and attachments.

Prompts are those predictable behaviors, events, ideas, or feelings that presently elicit the symptom. For Barbara, the pre-medical student who presented for pain control, the onset of her menstrual cycle had become a prompt for the occurrence of inordinate pain and accompanying feelings of frustration. For a cigarette smoker, the prompt might be the end of a meal, getting into his car, or drinking coffee. The symptom or behavior has become an automatic response to the prompt and, in this way, poses a challenge to any effort to eliminate that response. The symptom has, in essence, become a "solution" to the prompt.

When identifying and utilizing prompts in your suggestions, you are affirming the client's experience. They intimately know of their pain, urge to smoke, or depressive mood, and by reflecting that symptom in your suggestion, you establish immediate rapport and enhance the therapeutic alliance. In this way, the inclusion of prompts establishes a stepping-stone to additional therapeutic suggestions encompassing the use of cues and attachments.

Hypnotic suggestions need not avoid these prompts. Rather, the prediction of them will further validate the accuracy of the suggestion and avoid resistance in the process. The purpose of hypnosis is to alter the response, not the prompt. Barbara was able to uncover the purpose of her symptom and construct a healthier response. The smoker might be taught to be more vigilant to his prompts and to replace the cigarette with a more desirable response.

Cues are the beliefs, emotions, and/or habituated sensory responses that accompany the prompts. For Barbara it was the belief that she could not function because her pain inhibited her. When the smoker feels the urge for a cigarette, he might experience a feeling in his mouth, the thought that "it's time for a cigarette," or an emotional state such as anger or sadness. Thus, a suggestion stating, "At the first signs of your period, whether it be a feeling of being bloated, indigestion, or some other indication (prompt), you can remember that as a mature woman, you have a wonderful biological system which can manage this normal event with ease, allowing you to use your energy and intelligence for more important and interesting endeavors" (cue). To the smoker, it could be suggested, "Whenever you feel that old sensation to pick up a cigarette (prompt), you will automatically begin to breathe full, deep breaths" (cue).

Attachments are the outcomes that you hope to connect to the previously troublesome events that have supported the symptom. Thus, with Barbara the addition of the suggestion, "and you can be curious to see just how many luxurious baths and steamy novels you will enjoy during this time of physical renewal." The smoker can be reminded of the many reasons that he has for becoming free of cigarettes, such as, "and with each breath you feel more and more in control, anticipating the many happy times ahead with your grandchildren."

The weaving of attachments, cues, and prompts into suggestions has a basis both in Erickson's encouraging the development of a "Yes Set" (Erickson et al., 1976) with a client, and in the pacing and leading of suggestions as described earlier in this text. Erickson illustrated that a client's cooperation was heightened by "priming the pump," that is, asking a series of questions for which the obvious answer was "yes." Not unlike the game of follow-the-leader, one becomes accustomed to responding in a particular way. As shown earlier, pacing suggestions has a similar effect, since it encourages the client along a certain cognitive pathway. The leading suggestion then has an increased chance of success. Therapeutic suggestions that follow these guidelines are embraced with little resistance.

In delineating these three elements of suggestion — prompts, cues, and attachments — we hope to make more accessible and practical their use in creating successful suggestions.

WORST-CASE SCENARIOS: ABREACTIONS AND IDIOSYNCRATIC RESPONSES

Regardless of how comfortable and familiar they might feel with clients and their diagnostic picture, many therapists fear that hypnosis could precipitate uncontrollable abreaction in fragile clients. Although abreactions do occur with the use of hypnosis, they are relatively rare and often less dramatic than anticipated. We will address therapists' concerns regarding abreactions as well as techniques for managing them.

That being said, dramatic situations can and do occur with the use of hypnosis. When working with Paula for her chronic insomnia, I (RV) was giving her the typical suggestions for peaceful, pleasant imagery and asking for an ideomotor signal to indicate when she attained this experience. Nothing happened. I added, "Take all the time you need...," and still nothing happened. So, I asked, "What's happening?" No response. I continued, "Who are you?" She said, "Nobody." "Where are you?" "Nowhere...I am dead." Okay, well, at least I knew she was not asleep. Otherwise, I was totally surprised and mystified by this turn of events with a woman whom I thought I knew quite well.

Another week, Paula surprised me once again. I had reoriented her following trance work that targeted trance management — that is, being able to control her depth and maintain contact with me — I thought, successfully. When I left my office an hour later after my last client, I found her sitting on the floor at the other end of my long hallway, in a fetal position. I asked her to come with me and we returned to my office. She was clearly already in a trance. In fact, she had never fully reoriented from trance. Eventually, it became apparent that I had made contact with a dissociative identity disorder in a client I had known for years. While initially frightening, this became a very productive phase of treatment. Ironically, after these sessions, she reported sleeping and feeling better than she had in weeks, although she was not sure why.

Although I had treated Paula over the course of several years for poor self-esteem due to childhood abuse, relationship issues, and, later, marital and parenting issues, I had just stumbled upon a new dimension to her psychological makeup. Paula had revealed to me a dissociative identity disorder that had previously escaped our recognition. Our work, both hypnotic and otherwise, took a more productive direction. Thus, the behaviors that initially startled me provided an opportunity for my therapy with Paula to take a new and more profound path.

In another instance, when using the standard staircase technique for deepening, my (RV) middle-aged female client began to weep. Once again, being a relatively novice hypnotherapist, I was unnerved. I ultimately rallied, suggesting she would understand her tears to a degree and with as much emotion as she was prepared for at that time. Upon reorienting, she informed me that, at age six, she was walking down the stairs when she learned of her mother's death. Prior to this hypnotic imagery, she had not recalled this detail.

It is likely that most abreactive and unexpected experiences occur with trauma survivors, but not exclusively. First, we do not know for sure if our clients have suffered trauma. Secondly, what might seem to be benign images to us could evoke disturbing associations for them. I discovered this possibility early in my (MD) hypnosis career when working with Nancy. Knowing that she grew up on a farm, I innocently suggested that she recall a warm summer day in the fields. Quite unexpectedly, she began hyperventilating. During our discussions of her family history, she had failed to mention that her younger brother had wandered into the road on such a day and was struck by a car and killed. It is important to add that, although this recollection was unanticipated and startling, it was nevertheless fortuitous in directing the course of treatment.

Again, the hypnotherapist is called upon to overcome performance anxiety and be creative. One of my (RV) supervisors relieved my feelings of confusion and failure by stressing (often), "Remember that you're a good, seasoned therapist. Treat your client, and your client is the unconscious." Rather than feeling I needed to do magic, I learned to simply rely on my therapeutic skills. If we find ourselves suddenly with a sad six-year-old, we treat a sad six-year-old.

This point was brought home to us at a recent workshop. Dr. Voit was conducting a demonstration with one of the participants and, as sometimes happens, other participants also went into trance. Suddenly Janice, sitting two seats away from me (MD), began shaking and sobbing: "I can't get out! I can't get out! My hands are so cold!" Moving to her side, I asked Janice if I could hold her hands. When she agreed, I took her hands and told her to feel the warmth of mine coming into hers. I then asked her to tell me whether she could feel my hands holding hers. She said that she could. "Good," I said. "Feeling my hands means you are not alone, right?" Head nod. "And you don't know yet which of your hands will get the warmest." Janice gradually reoriented to her surroundings and expressed her own surprise at what had occurred. Dr. Voit's demonstration with another student had evoked a repressed memory that she had believed to be sufficiently addressed. It is our understanding that Janice returned to therapy for a more complete resolution to her conflicts.

Although this spontaneous regression did not occur in a psycho-therapy context, it was nonetheless an abreaction. You may not have a clue as to what the nature of the reaction might be, but you would nonetheless respond to the client not as someone lost in an abnormal experience, but as you normally would. The first thing Janice needed to know was that she was not alone and that she would be okay. This was accomplished by helping her to reorient to her presence at our workshop, to who I was and that I could help her, and, of course, to the present date. Lastly, she needed to know that she could manage her experience now and in the future. As we later processed these events, Dr. Voit made the observation that I had reacted not as a hypnotherapist but as a therapist. Although I might be reluctant to take a client's hands under normal conditions, when a client is in need of immediate "grounding," this is an option to be considered. Otherwise, all my other interventions were variations of what most therapists would do under similar circumstances.

TREATMENT PLANNING: APPLICATIONS

Although it is a bit of an overgeneralization, it is rare that our clients do not enter therapy without some degree of depression or anxiety.

In this context, we use the term "depression" to describe feelings of helplessness, immobility, low energy, and impoverished ego strength. By anxiety, we are referring to emotional hypervigilance, preoccupation with the future, and, of course, physiological tension and arousal. Therefore, we are going to address hypnotic treatment planning for these symptoms in the belief that these guidelines might create a foundation from which to work. Needless to say, the specifics of your language will be heavily influenced by each of your clients.

For both depression and anxiety, we provide tables below that translate symptoms into hypnotic phenomena and, then, what interventions might be indicated by these phenomena.

Depression and Helplessness

Depressive Symptoms and Hypnotic Phenomena
As any therapist can attest, those suffering from depression can be among our most difficult and frustrating clients. We know that chemical depression and dysthymia are usually not responsive to psychotherapy alone and will likely benefit from psychotropic medication. Those with situational, chronic depression are generally negative, have low motivation, and feel hopeless that anyone or anything can help. As psychotherapists, we have become familiar with the "learned helplessness" phenomenon whereby one who has been unable to escape pain eventually gives up any attempt to do so. Such a belief becomes deeply internalized and prevents movement or change.

Perhaps it is because of the negativity and helplessness that exemplify depression that many of our peers consider hypnosis to be contraindicated in its treatment. Because these clients are not expecting a positive experience or success, they will present with considerable resistance. Any intervention that elicits doubt or even hope could be defeated before it has a chance to be proven beneficial.

Yet we maintain that depressed clients can benefit from the use of hypnosis when they are assessed in appropriate, hypnotic terms. Depression could be considered a form of natural trance (catalepsy, anesthesia) and an absorption into pessimism and crippling emotional pain. The success of treatment will be a result of the use of appropriate language, the accurate interpretation of symptoms into hypnotic talents, and the corresponding utilization of these phenomena in the process of treatment planning.

Carrie initially sought treatment (RV) for weight loss. Although she only wanted to lose 40 pounds, she felt miserable with her body and described herself as "obese." She admitted that she avoided life's conflicts and naively hoped that hypnosis would provide the magical, uncomplicated solution she needed. The introduction of a simple food diary, where she would make note of everything she ate or drank, did provide improved self-awareness and a gradual weight loss that created hope and renewed confidence. Carrie lost 20 pounds — and then hit a wall. She stopped losing weight, stopped taking her long walks, and was again disgusted and despondent. This personal impasse was reflected in her therapy, as nothing seemed to help and her interest was waning.

As is often the case with overweight people, Carrie was detached from her physical and emotional experience. She was as disconnected from hunger and fullness as she was from the sadness and frustration that characterized both her family and marital relationships. As her pain grew over the years, so did her need to repress and deny. She was "cut off" at the neck and rigidly guarded against any attempts to reach beyond her defenses.

Essentially, Carrie was depressed and without hope. Viewed hypnotically, she was cataleptic (immobile and inflexible), dissociated (from hunger and fullness), anesthetic (unable and unwilling to feel painful emotions), age regressed (reliant upon childhood adaptation to neglect), both negatively (ignoring attention and nurturing) and positively (imagining disapproval) hallucinating, and experiencing time distortion (her depressed moods could seem endless). Hypnosis would need to embrace these talents, from induction through the offering of post-hypnotic induction, in order to gain Carrie's absorption and focus and to engage and move her from the depths of her depression.

In Table 7.1, we again demonstrate the "translation" of symptoms common with depressed clients and the hypnotic phenomena that will become the focal points of your hypnotic treatment planning:

Language and the Hypnotic Relationship
Once you have assessed your client in hypnotic terms, certain implications for your language and hypnotic relationship begin to emerge. With any client, you have to begin with "where she's at" and lead her to a healthier place. While some clients are motivated and trusting enough to allow you to work against their hypnotic talents, depressed individuals need to be met in their misery. It is like lifting a heavy object: You will be more successful and exert less strain if you get under that object, not lift it from the top. With the depressed client,

Table 7.1

Depressive symptoms	Hypnotic phenomena
Low motivation and energy	Catalepsy
Flat affect	Dissociation
	Anesthesia
Helplessness	Time expansion
	Negative hallucination
	Age regression
Negativity	Positive hallucination
Appetite changes	Dissociation

this strategy also aids in trust, as your empathy will feel genuine and accurate. Furthermore, you will also bypass the considerable resistance that we mentioned earlier.

The seeding of ideas in your waking-state interactions must be both encouraging and respectful of your client's helplessness. In a sense, you are beginning treatment with ego enhancement in hopes of eliciting some degree of assistance and cooperation from her. I (RV) view antidepressant medication as comparable to a jack is used in changing a tire. It is very difficult to remove and replace a flat tire without one. We still have to sweat and get our hands dirty, but the jack will raise the car enough to make the work easier. Once the tire is changed, we no longer have need for the jack and we can safely drive away. Such is the early goal of therapy and hypnosis for depression. It is the lifting off the ground that makes "change" more manageable.

As we suggested earlier, many of the words often used in hypnotic language are not indicated in treating depression. We do not want to suggest "down...heavy...deeper" to someone who has been unable to pull herself up from overwhelming burdens and hopelessness. Instead, we would suggest using words such as "further" and "lighter" to describe the experience of trance depth. Furthermore, we want to encourage connectedness, not dissociation. In small steps, the depressed client needs to reconnect with the very emotions that had become so paralyzing. As you can likely see, becoming mindful of these considerations will lay the groundwork for later interventions.

Hypnotic Phenomena and Treating Depression
Table 7.2 suggests how the hypnotic phenomena common with depression correspond to hypnotic interventions:

My hypnotic inductions with Carrie began with involuntary eye closure and arm levitation in order to utilize her talent for dissociation.

Table 7.2

Hypnotic phenomena	Treatment strategies
Catalepsy	Movement imagery
	Trance ratification provides sense of autonomy, efficacy, and control
	Challenging rigid, self-destructive belief systems
Dissociation	Connecting parts
	Metaphors about integration
	Reinforcing positive ego states
Negative hallucination	Seeing things with "new eyes"
	Ego enhancement
Positive hallucination	Metaphors about correcting distortions
	Redefining negative memory and perception
Time expansion	Metaphors about here and now, positive future
	Movement imagery
Amnesia	Positive affect bridge
	Ego enhancement
Hypermnesia	Letting-go imagery
Hypersensitivity	Shield imagery
	Providing means of managing negative affect and emotional states
Age regression	Post-hypnotic suggestion for present focus
	Re-nurturing
	Redefining negative memory and perception
	Facilitating a curative self-nurturing experience
	Future self-orientation
Anesthesia	Ability to control emotion

As she became more trusting and relaxed with hypnosis, I began to lead her toward an improved body awareness with simple internal focused absorption and attention to breathing. I deepened her trance with essentially more of the same, concentrating on her internal experience and natural connectedness. Thus, by the time Carrie was comfortably, deeply hypnotized, I had already initiated my intervention.

During the course of treatment, I presented various images to Carrie. Themes of locating and reinforcing strength, movement, and integration continued throughout. There were indirect suggestions of new insight and a growing awareness and tolerance for her repressed emotions and needs. For several sessions, she visited herself as a child, offering nurturance and words of wisdom. I made tapes of such themes for her use at home, and she eventually learned to practice self-hypnosis without them.

Gradually, Carrie began to emerge from her self-protective cata-lepsy. She discovered anger, which grew into healthy assertiveness. She discovered sadness, which grew into self-understanding and enti-tlement. These recovered and renovated facets allowed her to seek changes in her marriage, work, and lifestyle. As her life began to move, so did she. Carrie ate a conscious and self-nurturing diet. Again she walked and pounds disappeared. Although she at times reported dis-tress and displeasure with her existence, she appreciated the value of emotional range and the direction that emotions provided.

There was no single image or intervention that relieved Carrie's depression. Rather, it was the way in which we embraced and utilized her condition in hypnotic terms. Her unconscious processes were altered, not removed. With continued therapeutic supervision and an occasional gentle nudge, Carrie continues to carry herself forward.

Anxiety

Anxiety Symptoms and Hypnotic Phenomena
I (RV) recently met with a new client who was told by her primary care physician that anxiety is "like an allergy. Some people just end up getting it." We often forget how many individuals, highly educated or not, do not understand how the human body functions. Therefore, any treatment of anxiety disorders should begin by providing an edu-cation about the nature of these symptoms — that they comprise an adaptive physiological response to perceived danger. Anxiety is what the body does to survive external threats of harm. Therefore, prior to beginning hypnotherapy, our clients must be taught that the rapid heartbeat, the short, tight breathing, the rush of adrenaline, and the light-headedness are all normal and protective. When these symptoms are presented to us for psychotherapy, the dangers are usually merely perceived, imagined, or internally generated. The inability to attach these physical responses to a real danger is what magnifies clients' fear and a belief they are losing control.

We are assuming that this "waking-state reframing" of their anx-iety experience is, in some ways, reassuring to the conscious and unconscious dread that has become habituated. Our experience has been that, at the very least, it certainly helps to eliminate the secondary fears that one is losing total control or suffering a heart attack. In a sense, we have also accomplished two additional goals.

By connecting anxiety symptoms to a natural, unconscious pro-cess, we are handing the responsibility for these symptoms to our clients. This acceptance of responsibility will create an inescapable and desired paradox. If anxiety is both internally generated and instinctively protective, the sufferer cannot truly be losing control. Furthermore, if he owns the responsibility for his symptoms, and control is within his grasp, he can begin to learn new means of managing symptoms and finding relief.

I (RV) have often compared human anxiety and panic to the function of a smoke alarm. If there is a fire, the alarm alerts us to the emergency. On other occasions, the smoke from a boiling pot of water can unnecessarily set off the loud screech. Once we realize that there is no fire, we can reset the alarm and go back to what we were doing. The alarm warned us as it was supposed to, but it was mistaken. If only humans had a reset button that could quickly eliminate unwarranted symptoms. Such is the nature of hypnotherapy for anxiety. Our goal is to teach the client's unconscious about the source of the origin of his symptoms, that he can control those symptoms, and that one can learn new, healthier ways of responding to the precipitating factors.

Robert was a young man who had graduated with a degree in art education and looked forward to success as a teacher and painter. Unfortunately, job opportunities had been few and he was forced into a government office job. He initially believed this course to be temporary, but college loans and the financial needs of his new family prevented him from leaving. He did well and actually advanced in this profitable yet accidental career.

One afternoon, Robert believed he was having a heart attack. His father had suffered one, so he knew the signs: chest pains that radiated down his arms, shortness of breath, and dizziness. He was taken to a nearby emergency room, where an EKG revealed no problems with his heart. Instead, his doctor diagnosed his symptoms as panic and recommended that he see a psychologist. But what would cause panic? He was sitting at his desk doing his work. Why then? Why now?

When Robert arrived at my (RV) office, he was tense and confused. While admitting that he had recently been more agitated than usual, he believed that he was content with his life and had never considered counseling. However, Robert had been sleeping restlessly in recent weeks and was experiencing occasional headaches and muscle tightness in his shoulders and neck. Most importantly to him, Robert was unable to focus on his painting, normally a passion that could consume an entire weekend.

Robert responded well to the suggestion of hypnosis, although he carried the usual misconceptions that it would involve some relinquishing of control. These concerns were relieved by my usual education about hypnosis and a brief, successful relaxation exercise. In beginning hypnotherapy, my induction would start with Robert's strengths. While anxiety does involve dissociation, I would instead go with his close attention to his physiological state. In other words, I would *encourage* a focused absorption into his muscle tension, heartbeat, breathing, and hypervigilance to stimuli. Initially, I would not promote relaxation or any suggestion that he let go of control. In this way, I seized upon his preoccupation with sensation (hypersthesia) and sense of immediacy (time condensation). To deepen his trance, I encouraged him to anticipate what was about to happen and how it might feel, thus utilizing his fixation on future events (age progression). As indicated by Robert's artistic talents, my suggestions were laced with visual imagery throughout the induction and deepening of trance.

As it turned out, Robert was quite responsive to hypnosis. While creativity is considered to be a correlate of hypnotizability, we believe it is the utilization of hypnotic phenomena that broadens the access to trance and sidesteps the potential barriers implicit with anxiety disorders.

Table 7.3 demonstrates the "translation" of symptoms common with anxious or panicked clients and the hypnotic phenomena that will become the focal points of your hypnotic treatment planning:

Table 7.3

Anxiety symptoms	Hypnotic phenomena
Fear and apprehension	Age progression
Preoccupation with physical experience	Hypersthesia
Sense of immediacy	Time condensation
Perceived loss of control	Fluidity/flexibility
Reactivity to stimuli	Association
Fear of repeating past episodes	Hypermnesia
Panic	Catalepsy
Perceived loss of control	Dissociation

Language and the Hypnotic Relationship
For clients such as Robert, the idea of hypnosis might also evoke mistaken fears of losing control. The mere suggestion of relaxation, "letting go" of their protective physical tension, can be met with resistance and failure. Such words might also inhibit rapport, as the therapist could be unconsciously perceived as a threat to safety. For these reasons, we prefer to pace and lead our anxious clients. While learning to relax will be the critical aspect of their treatment, it is not the best place to begin.

As demonstrated with Robert, we prefer to begin by engaging the symptoms, which is another way of saying that we utilize hypnotic talents. While you will not want your language to reflect the heaviness and helplessness of the depressed client, we are proposing that you do embrace the tension and hypervigilance common with anxiety. In fact, it is sometimes even helpful to first suggest an *increase* in his symptoms prior to offering relief. This practice provides powerful trance-ratification benefits and begins the pacing and leading process.

When you have engaged your client with attention to his anxiety symptoms, you can then use his focused attention to introduce relaxation. Most therapists are familiar with the concept of *reciprocal inhibition* (Hall & Lindzey, 1957). In the most simplistic terms, we cannot be in two places at once. For our purposes, a person cannot be simultaneously tense and relaxed. Thus, when your client learns to notice the difference and that he can consciously make this choice, his recovery is well under way. Making note of the contrast and even alternating his experience from relaxed to anxious and back, such fractionation deepens the trance and teaches an invaluable unconscious lesson. You will gradually begin to concentrate on "learning" to relax and offering post-hypnotic suggestions for its natural occurrence.

We place the word "learning" in quotation marks because relaxation is, theoretically, our natural state of being. Because of our belief systems and life events, our bodies become habitually reactive and alerted. The corresponding chemistry and physiology establish a baseline condition that is anything but relaxed. Using an automobile metaphor, our engines are "idling" high most of the time. Yet we believe it is easier and perhaps more natural to recover a client's relaxation skills by referring to his natural ones. Similar to our ego-enhancement suggestions in our "Wonderment as the Beginning of Wisdom" section, we refer back to the many times a client has been relaxed, such as lying almost asleep in bed, swinging in a hammock on a pleasant afternoon, or sitting by the ocean watching or listening to the waves. These are experiences almost all of us have had, and their recollection will serve to reciprocally inhibit anxiety.

My approach with Robert was to direct his attention to internal cognitive and physiological activity, speaking rather quickly at first. When he began to exhibit trance behavior, I gradually softened and slowed my speech and refocused his attention to the first signs of relaxation. His existing anticipation was utilized into "curiosity," "interest," and "pleasant surprise." He was led into a deepened state of relaxation, while being given full control and choice. My suggestions for relaxation were all qualified with, "to whatever extent you find comfortable...no less...and no more." Similarly, I reinforced a here-and-now orientation that would calm his apprehensions and assure his trust in future, more provocative imagery. After only a few sessions, Robert began to appear more confident and receptive to hypnosis. It was time to begin further intervention.

Hypnotic Phenomena and Treating Anxiety

Once again, in Table 7.4, we offer suggestions for treatment strategies that might correspond to the hypnotic talents of the anxious client:

Table 7.4

Hypnotic phenomena	Treatment strategies
Time condensation	Imagery about time progressing
	Seeing the "big picture"
	Trance experience itself is usually a source of relaxation and relief from anxiety
Age progression	Metaphors about "here and now"
	Creation of positive future orientation in anxiety-provoking situations
Hypersensitivity	Detachment
	Utilizing inability to be in two places at one time, i.e., reciprocal inhibition
Fluidity/flexibility	Trance ratification
	Relaxation/breathing
	Increasing overall ego strength
Association	Boundary imagery
Hypermnesia	Here-and-now imagery
	Initially used to access past positive experiences
	Increasing a sense of efficacy by managing negative affects
Catalepsy	Movement imagery
	Increasing overall ego strength
Dissociation	Suggestions for insight, answers

Because Robert had been responsive to my early utilization of symptom-evident hypnotic phenomena and had become eager to include hypnosis in his treatment, I was able to make use of his talent for dissociation by introducing more trance-ratifying inductions. A simple involuntary eye closure and the Chaisson arm drop technique demonstrated for Robert the potential of his unconscious to control symptoms.

With these accomplishments as landmarks, I introduced ego-strength-ening suggestions that I would continue throughout treatment.

This theme was further built upon with an affect bridge to positive memories of accomplishment and self-control. Suggestions were made that he could become fixated on the strength experienced in these memories (utilizing his talents for catalepsy and hypermnesia) and bring them forward in time to the present. From that point, we maintained a here-and-now, "all the time you need" focus to counter his propensities for time progression and time condensation. Finally, I introduced guided imagery and indirect post-hypnotic suggestions where he might start with a blank canvas and begin to construct a painting that would reveal the meaning of and solutions to his symptoms.

It was not long before Robert had created a painting of his desk and a large window. He realized what might have been obvious to others: that he was trapped in a workplace ill-suited for his personality and that he yearned for a lifestyle more appropriate to his artistic expression. He had learned and effectively used relaxation skills to control anxiety and gained the necessary ego strength to confront the situation from which they had emerged. Yet it was this realization that led to an elementary school art teaching position that would construc-tively alter that situation and, hopefully, prevent further episodes.

There is one further point we want to make regarding the treat-ment of anxious clients. It is our belief that uncovering the origins and precipitants of current symptoms can be important. However, given the reciprocal inhibition premise, we do not believe it is always nec-essary. In Robert's case, it was, because it led to a major life decision. In other situations, the harnessing of physiological states will suffice in preventing further problems with major anxiety.

Years ago, I (MD) was asked to give a presentation at a suburban hospital. A few months prior to the invitation, I had interviewed to obtain privileges at this same hospital. The medical director had been impressed that I worked with geriatric clients and inquired if I would do a two-hour presentation entitled "Communicating with the Elderly Patient." I made it clear that I was not an expert on the topic, but that I would be glad to share what knowledge I had. A few days before the presentation, I heard from a colleague who provides services to stroke victims at a different facility. She called to say she would be attending the presentation. It was then I learned that this presentation had been marketed to numerous retirement community directors, rehabilitation providers, and nursing-home personnel in the area. I panicked. I was no expert! As a result, I developed such a case of stage fright that I struggled just to finish my lecture notes. Fortunately, I knew enough about cognitive distortions to eventually realize that it was unlikely the crowd would really throw tomatoes at me or walk out in droves.

We hope that you have not become so immobilized by performance anxiety with the integration of hypnosis into your practice. As with my presentation, most of our anxiety arises from the belief that we are going to fail or even make fools of ourselves. My anxiety diminished once I took the focus off of myself and placed it on my audience. I realized that I had the good fortune, not misfortune, to be addressing many of the area's experienced geriatric care providers. By emphasizing this stellar group's active expertise and participation, I was practically assured of an interesting and successful presentation. We believe that, by making a similar shift in focus away from yourself and onto your client, you will also relieve many of your apprehensions and discover the integration of hypnosis to be virtually effortless.

The constructs and treatment guidelines presented in this chapter are done so in an intentionally simplistic fashion. There are many other publications available that can offer a far more comprehensive coverage of these topics, and we urge our readers to make full use of the well-researched information that they provide. After we had included much of this material in a recent workshop on treatment planning, one student said to us, "This pulled it all together for me." We are hoping that you will have such a positive response and that the integration of hypnosis into your work will be a more natural and rewarding experience.

CHAPTER 8

Looking Forward to Looking Back

I (RV) was only seven when Santa brought me my very first guitar. It was a Martin guitar and, even at that young age, I knew I had the absolute best. My older brother was my early musical mentor and teacher, as he had already begun strumming his Gibson and singing the Top 40 hits we heard on the radio. He was taller, cooler, and a teenager. His influence was subtle but sure, and I suppose that, at the time, I wanted to be like him.

It was sometime during the next year that he and I, dressed in coats and clip-on ties, performed two hymns at our Baptist church Sunday evening prayer meeting. My focus was squarely on the instrumental accompaniment my stubby little seven-year-old fingers were hoping to articulate. I can no longer recall the actual performance, only that I had broken my E string that morning and was very, very nervous. I do know that, although it would take me years to appreciate, some part of me changed that day. Following my brother's lead, I began to transcend my struggling childhood identity. From that point, my "what makes me think I can do this?" became "what makes me think I can't?"

Here was a kid who had been too bashful to square dance in the elementary school auditorium or to read aloud in class. I was so quiet that my first-grade teacher sat me next to Shirley, the chattiest girl in our room. Low self-confidence had also inhibited my efforts in athletics, thus relegating me for years to the last to be chosen. But, somehow, my musical career began much differently. I must have been walking in my brother's wake to become so unimpressed with my own anxieties and shyness. I was still socially withdrawn, clumsy at sports, and my fingers were still stubby. Yet, for whatever reason, my guitar helped me dare to step across that juncture where fear meets excitement. I also discovered I was talented and that it was just fine to let others know.

Soon came the warm summer days when my neighborhood friends would watch through the screen door as my brother and I practiced our interpretations of Elvis Presley and Ricky Nelson. He was Elvis and I was important merely to be playing with Elvis. I enjoyed the attention while stiffening from the pressure to impress my peers. One member of our admiring audience, Barbara, soon became my childhood sweetheart and best friend for years to come. As many children will do, she and I would stage regular talent shows in her basement and charge a small admission for those lacking the talent or guts to take part. My recollection is that she would dance or dress up her dog Deedee and I would play my guitar. Barbara was the most loyal and relentless friend I've ever had. She seemed to like and enjoy everything I did. In sharing so much of myself with her and having it appreciated and affirmed, I guess I began to trust who I was becoming and I liked him.

Years later, a high school friend and drummer asked if I would like to audition for a fledgling rock band boldly named "the Gladiators." Uh, sure. Like in many loosely formed teenage ensembles, there were already several guitarists. Upon my first meeting Bernie, the group's self-anointed leader, he said, "You can leave your guitar at home. We need a singer." Until that point, my brother had been the singer. My vocal talents had only involved the school chorus and singing tenor to ear-splitting renditions of show tunes. I can recall my grandmother humming gospel melodies and my mother teaching me harmonies to our early 45s. Still, I had never considered myself to be a vocalist.

Once again, I felt the fear. Once again, I said, "Uh, sure."

Now I was a guitarist *and* a lead singer. I could stand in front of large groups of strangers and bellow lyrics into a microphone. People would dance to my music. For the most part, I became increasingly comfortable with the risk and exposure required to be a church-dance rock star. The exceptions were times when family or friends would attend our shows. There was something uncomfortably intimate about sharing my new persona with people who knew me otherwise. The same has always been true with playing and singing in a living room or one-on-one. Perhaps the scrutiny is too great as my audience of one casts her focused absorption on me. It leaves much too much room for error and embarrassment, the dreaded artifacts of my pre-musical identity.

As the reader is already aware, I never became a celebrity. I did, however, manage a part-time musical career that introduced me to many interesting people and a great deal of fun. Throughout my high school and early college years, my band performed the Beatles, Buddy Holly, and even "soul" music. Upon discovering that I was a hippie, I joined Jean, a blond-haired songstress, to mimic the sounds of Peter, Paul and Mary, Donovan, and Dylan at coffeehouses and outdoor concerts. After college, I formed a trio to earn a little extra spending money at drinking establishments. Following in the country-rock trend of the early seventies, we performed songs by John Prine and the Eagles with the addition of a few original compositions. Over the years I had been performing, there seemed to be an interactive effect between the breadth of my repertoire and my comfort on stage that began to feel more and more like "home." The more I knew, the more natural it felt. The more natural it felt, the more I knew.

While I was in graduate school, much to the dare of an amused housemate, I auditioned as a solo act at the Mousetrap, one of my favorite haunts. I prepared three or four numbers, expecting to hear a simple "thanks, but no thanks." I played with tense (no longer stubby) fingers and tight vocal cords. But, as I departed the stage, the Mousetrap manager asked, "Can you play next Tuesday?" This shocking offer sent me into a spontaneous trance of panic and excitement. After recovering my composure, I managed a weak but audible, "Uh, sure." In less than a week, I would need nearly three hours of music, not three songs. I was being thrust into a new arena, my "home court" in a sense, no longer partially disguised and protected by my band, Jean, or a trio. What to do! Well, I did the only thing I knew how to do. I did the Beatles, Buddy Holly, PP&M, Dylan, and the Eagles.

For the next three years I performed solo at many of Charlottesville's smaller venues. Graced with reasonable talent and comfortably surrounded by the familiar works of my idols, the stage had become a second home. I even eventually found the courage to reveal my own compositions, which were usually based on personal experiences. Once again stepping across that juncture from fear to excitement, I discovered great satisfaction in disclosing these various facets of myself. It felt like a final step in the transformation as all I had learned and all that I was became one.

I have now been a practicing psychologist for over 20 years. In my bedroom sits one of my many guitars resting patiently against its stand. Every once in a while, sometimes more often, I pick it up and play. I will sing to myself and, on rare occasion, to my friends. Even as I become rusty, my fingers always remember where to go and what to do. Whether or not I am playing or singing, I know one thing. I *am* a musician.

We believe that just about anyone, indeed, every one of you...and that other *you* who learns, whether you are aware of it or not...can operate on many different levels at once.... And the you that is reading this can do so comfortably, knowing that nothing else is really important right now. That this moment is a moment when many things are possible.... And you can rest in the knowledge that you possess many talents, some which you tend to forget until the occasion arises to use them....

So in the matter of functioning autonomously on many levels simultaneously, you know that you already know how to make your bed while planning your day...or how to speak with a client while imagining her potentials...or even how to read while also not reading, but rather listening, and commenting to yourself about what a part of you is reading...while the listener listens and also comments or waits to hear more...and why not just listen? And follow wherever the words take you....

So that perhaps one day, you will find that
          a client will appear...
                    and without a second thought
          you understand
          she has developed certain talents...
Perhaps she knows how to forget
          or how to remember with exquisite detail
Perhaps she has developed the ability to stay so still in her life
          she has become immobilized....

Or perhaps she jumps so rapidly from one thought or feeling to
    the next
        that she is in perpetual confusion...
And imagine you realize that you are forward, looking back
        recalling when you felt the excitement of discovery
                That is amazing!
                How do they do that?
                        I want to be able to do that!
And the *that* is hypnosis
        Learning
        wanting to learn
        wanting to know how to create
        those wondrous experiences and new realities...
Maybe it seemed magical or almost mysterious
Perhaps you saw a demonstration subject
        experience catalepsy
        hallucinations
        relief of pain
Or perhaps you yourself did...
        witnessing one way or the other
        how good those feelings could be
        Time and space suspended...
And, like Prometheus capturing fire
        you wanted that light
        that spark
        those skills or that magic...
So you undertook a journey
        Like so many explorers do
        To find and capture
                that light
                that spark
                to become that healer
                you have dreamed of becoming...
Not realizing perhaps that as your journey progressed
                you would be
                challenged
                tested
                perhaps scorned
And from whence would the greatest challenges emerge?
        From within?
        Or from without?

Would the "wise" elders caution about the perils of fire
    Uncontrollable
    Hot
    Destructive
    The domain of the devil...
Or would the ghosts of prior failures
      provide your greatest challenges
      "Hubris cometh before the fall"
      Just who do you think you are anyway?
      What makes you think you can do this?
      Even if you try, you will fail miserably
      You will look a fool...
After all, curious Pandora did the forbidden...
      She opened the box
      Disgorging its horrific contents
      Thus, defiling a perfect world
      Aghast, mortified
      Sick of heart
She slammed the lid shut.
Only to be tormented further...
      A tiny voice,
      at first no more than a whisper
      Pleading
      Let me out!
      Please! Let me out!
So sweet a sound, so earnest an appeal
      but already so much to fear...
Fretfully relenting
      she lifted the cover,
      And out sprang
         Hope...
Courage rarely precedes action
It usually is the other way around
      The wish to be more
      To attain one's heart's desire,
      To risk when still in fear,
      This is how the spark is captured
      and tamed
      to bring forth
      the light you seek to share with others...

Conquering darkness
illuminating a new way
of being...
And they, like your Self
Will find their fears as merely
pebbles to be kicked away
not the eternal boulders they feared
Their courage to be found when needed
And their guide to be wise enough
to reveal the way...
So as you...
in your future
encounter these gifted individuals
you can rest in the knowledge
that they, too, will have a time
when they can look forward
to looking back.

References

American Psychological Association (2003). Ethical principles of psychologists and code of conduct. www.apa.org; retrieved February 28, 2003.

American Society of Clinical Hypnosis. (2003). Code of conduct. www.asch.net; retrieved July 19, 2003.

Anderson, P. *Magnolia*. With Philip Baker Hall, Julianne Moore, and Jason Robards. Screenplay: Paul Thomas Anderson. New Line Cinema, 1999.

Armstrong, G., dir. (1994). *Little Women*. With Wynona Ryder and Kirsten Dunst. Columbia/Tristar Studios.

Bandler, R., Grinder, J., & Delozier, J. (1977). *Patterns of the Hypnotic Techniques of Milton H. Erickson, M.D.* Volume I. Cupertino, CA: Meta Publications.

Barber, J. (1988). Naturalistic induction. In D. Hammond (Ed.), *Hypnotic induction & suggestion: An introductory manual*, Des Plaines, IL: American Society of Clinical Hypnosis.

Berra, Y., Kaplan, D., & Kaplan, D. (2001). *When you come to a fork in the road, take it!* New York: Hyperion.

Brown, D., & Fromm, E. (1986). *Hypnotherapy and Hypnoanalysis*. Hillsdale, NJ: Lawrence Erlbaum Associates.

Browne, J. For a dancer. On Jackson Browne, *Late for the sky*. Compact Disc. Electra/Asylum Records, 7E-1017-2.

Campbell, J. (1949). *The hero with a thousand faces*. Princeton, NJ: Princeton University Press.

Edgette, J., & Edgette, J. (1995). *The Handbook of Hypnotic Phenomena in Psychotherapy*. New York: Brunner/Mazel.

Erickson, M. (1954). Pseudo-orientation in time as a hypnotherapeutic procedure. *Journal of Clinical and Experiential Hypnosis, 2*, 261–283.

Erickson, M. (1958/1980). Naturalistic techniques of hypnosis. In Rossi, E (ed.), *The collected papers of Milton H. Erickson*. Volume I. New York: Irvington.

Erickson, M., & Ernest, R. (1989). *The February man: Evolving consciousness and identity in hypnosis*. New York: Brunner/Mazel.

Erickson, M., & Rossi, E. (1979). *Hypnotherapy*. New York: Irvington Publishing.

Erickson, M., Hershman, S., & Secter, I. (1981). *The practical application of medical and dental hypnosis: General medicine and dentistry, psychiatry, surgery, obstetrics and gynecology, anesthesiology, pediatrics.* Paperback edition. Seminars On Hypnosis Publishing Co.

Erickson, M., Rossi, E., & Rossi, S. (1976). *Hypnotic realities: The induction of clinical hypnosis and forms of indirect suggestion.* New York: Irvington Publishers.

Geary, B. (2001a). Assessment in Ericksonian hypnosis and psychotherapy. In B. B. Geary & J. K. Zeig (Eds.), *The handbook of Ericksonian psychotherapy.* Phoenix: The Milton H. Erickson Foundation Press.

Geary, B. (2001b). *Utilization of hypnotic phenomena in mind-body treatment.* American Society of Clinical Hypnosis Annual Meeting, Reno, NV.

Gilligan, S. G. (1987). *Therapeutic trances: The cooperation principle in Ericksonian hypnotherapy.* New York: Brunner/Mazel.

Grinder, J., Delozier, J., & Bandler, R. (1977). *Patterns of the hypnotic techniques of Milton H. Erickson, M.D.* Cupertino, CA: Meta Publications.

Grinder, J., & Bandler, R. (1981). *TRANCE-formation.* Moab, UT: Real People Press.

Haley, J. (1973). *Uncommon therapy: The psychiatric techniques of Milton Erickson, M.D.* New York: W. W. Norton & Company.

Hall, C. S., & Lindzey, G. (1957). *Theories of personality.* New York: John Wiley & Sons.

Hammond, D. (1988). *Hypnotic induction and suggestion: An introductory manual.* Des Plaines, IL: American Society of Clinical Hypnosis.

Hammond, D. (1990). *Handbook of hypnotic suggestions and metaphors.* New York: W. W. Norton & Company.

Hammond, D. et al. (1995). *Clinical hypnosis and memory: Guidelines for clinicians and for forensic hypnosis.* Des Plaines, IL: American Society of Clinical Hypnosis Press.

Hammond, D., & Cheek, D. (1988). Ideomotor Signaling: A method for rapid unconscious exploration. In Hammond, D. (ed.), *Hypnotic induction and suggestion: An introductory manual.* Des Plaines, IL: American Society of Clinical Hypnosis.

Hammond, D., & Elkins, G. (1994). *Standards of training in clinical hypnosis.* Des Plaines, IL: American Society of Clinical Hypnosis.

Havens, R. (1985). *The wisdom of Milton H. Erickson.* New York: Irvington Publishers.

Lankton, S., & Lankton, C. (1983). *The answer within: A clinical framework of Ericksonian hypnotherapy.* New York: Brunner/Mazel.

Levant, R. (2001). Desperately seeking language: Understanding, assessing and treating normative male alexithymia. In Brooks, G., & Good, G. (eds.), *The new handbook of counseling and psychotherapy for men.* Volume I. CA: Jossey-Bass.

Lucas, G., dir. (1977). *Star Wars.* With Mark Hammill, Harrison Ford, Carrie Fisher, and Alec Guinness. Screenplay: George Lucas. Lucasfilm.

Luhrmann, B., dir. (2002). *Moulin Rouge*. With Nicole Kidman, Ewan McGregor, and Jim Broadbent. Music Director: Marius DeVries. Twentieth Century Fox.

Mamet, D., dir. (1987). *House of Games*. With Joe Mantegna and Lindsay Crouse. Screenplay: Jonathan Katz and David Mamet. Orion.

Mayo, A., dir. (1931). *Svengali*. With John Barrymore, Marian Marsh, and Donald Crisp. Screenplay: J. Grubb Alexander. Troma Studios.

Mills, J., & Crowley, R. (1986). *Therapeutic metaphors for children and the child within*. New York: Brunner/Mazel.

Minuchin, S. (1974). *Families and family therapy*. Cambridge, MA: Harvard University Press.

Moore, Julianne. (2002). *Inside the actors studio*. Bravo Television Network. Host: James Lipton.

Moyers, B. (Executive editor) (1988). *Joseph Campbell and the power of myth with Bill Moyers*. [Television Series] New York: WNET; Chicago: WTTW.

Pearson, C. (1991). *Awakening the heroes within: Twelve archetypes to help us find ourselves and transform our world*. New York: HarperCollins.

Pert, Candace B. (1997). *Molecules of emotion*. New York: Scribner.

Reitman, I., dir. (1988). *Twins*. With Danny DeVito and Arnold Schwarzenegger. Screenplay: William Davies, William Osborne, Timothy Harris, and Herschel Weingrod. Universal.

Rossi, E., & Cheek, D. (1988). *Mind-body therapy: Methods of ideodynamic healing in hypnosis*. New York: W. W. Norton & Company.

Rossi, E. (1993). *The psychobiology of mind-body healing: New concepts of therapeutic hypnosis*. Revised Edition. New York: W. W. Norton & Company.

Rossi, E. (1996). *The symptom path to enlightenment: The new dynamics of self-organization in hypnotherapy: An advanced manual for beginners*. Edited by Kathryn Lane Rossi. Pacific Palisades, CA: Pacific Palisades Publishing.

Shor, R., & Orne, E. (1959). *The Harvard group scale of hypnotic susceptibility*. Palo Alto: Consulting Psychologists Press.

Society for Clinical and Experimental Hypnosis. (2001). The Society for Clinical and Experimental Hypnosis: Code of Ethics. *Membership Resource Directory: 2001*, 61–64.

Spiegel, H., & Spiegel, D. (1978). *Trance and treatment*. New York: Basic Books.

van der Kolk, B., McFarlane, A., & Weisaeth, L. (Eds.) (1996). *Traumatic stress: The effects of overwhelming experience on mind, body and society*. New York: Guilford.

Watkins, J. (1987). *Hypnotherapeutic techniques: The practice of clinical hypnosis*, Volume I, New York: Irvington Publishers.

Watzlavick, P., Weakland, J., & Fisch, R. (1974). *Change*. New York: W. W. Norton & Company.

Weitzenhoffer, A. (1989). *The practice of hypnotism: Traditional and semi-traditional techniques and phenomenology*. Volumes One and Two. New York: John Wiley & Sons.

Weitzenhoffer, A., & Hilgard, E. (1959). *Stanford hypnotic susceptibility scale, forms A and B*. Stanford, CA: Consulting Psychologists Press.

Wulf, R. (1996). The historical roots of Gestalt therapy theory. Gestalt Dialogue: *Newsletter for the Integrative Gestalt Centre*. (see Aoteatoa, New Zealand, Nov. 1996 edition.)

Yapko, M. (1994). *Essentials of hypnosis*. New York: Brunner/Mazel.

Yapko, M. (2003). *Trancework*. Third Edition. New York: Brunner-Routledge.

Zeig, J. (1980). *A teaching seminar with Milton H. Erickson*. New York: Brunner/Mazel.

APPENDIX A:

Professional Organizations

The American Society of Clinical Hypnosis
140 North Bloomingdale Road
Bloomingdale, IL 60108-1017
Phone: (630) 980-4740
Fax: (630) 351-8490
www.asch.net (with links to component and other organizations)
E-mail: info@asch.net

Society for Clinical and Experimental Hypnosis
Central Office
Washington State University
PO Box 642114
Pullman, WA 99164-2114
Phone: (509) 335-7504
Fax: (509) 335-2097
E-mail: sceh@wsu.edu

The Milton H. Erickson Foundation, Inc.
3606 North 24th Street
Phoenix, AZ 85016
(602) 956-6196
www.erickson-foundation.org

DeLaney & Voit, Inc.
Hypnosis Education and Consultation Resources
98 Maine Street
Brunswick, ME 04011
(207) 721-0500
www.delaneyandvoit.com
E-mail: delaneyandvoit@yahoo.com

Hypnotic Treatment Planning Worksheet

Diagnosis and Treatment Planning
Utilizing Hypnosis and Hypnotic Phenomena

Focal Problems: *Possible Purposes of Symptoms*

1. _____   1. _____
2. _____   2. _____
3. _____   3. _____

Hypnotic Phenomena Client Currently Exhibits

Dissociation   Connectiveness
Catalepsy   Fluidity/Flexibility
Age Regression   Age Progression
Amnesia   Hypermnesia
Anesthesia/Analgesia   Hypersensitivity
Time Expansion   Time Condensation

Sensory Strengths (Primary, Secondary, Tertiary)

Auditory _____   Visual _____   Tactile _____

Purpose of Resistance

Strategies for Utilizing the Resistance

Client's Metaphors and Images

Induction Strategies:

Goal of This Session:

Future Work:

APPENDIX C:

Informed Consent Form[1]

Sample Informed Consent Document

The Nature of Hypnosis. Memory is imperfect, whether or not hypnosis is used. Memory is not like a tape recorder, and rarely will all the details of any recollection be fully accurate. People have been shown to be capable of filling in gaps in memory, of distorting information, and of being influenced in what is "remembered" by leading questions or suggestions. For example, our memories may sometimes be influenced through reading, movies, TV, or conversations. Thus, research has shown that there is no guarantee that information remembered through hypnosis (or through ordinary recall) is factually accurate. On the other hand, information that is so remembered through hypnosis may in fact be accurate. But the only way one may know definitively whether something recalled under hypnosis is accurate is to obtain independent corroboration. Thus, if you should remember something under hypnosis, regard this information as simply one more source of data that cannot be relied on as more accurate or necessarily superior

[1] Reprinted with the permission of the American Society of Clinical Hypnosis Press. Originally printed in Hammond, D., & Elkins, G., *Standards of Training in Clinical Hypnosis*. Des Plaines, IL: American Society of Clinical Hypnosis, copyright 1994.

to material already in conscious awareness. Such further data would simply be information to be weighed and evaluated in therapy along with what you already consciously know.

Potential Legal Issues. In many jurisdictions, courts have held that a person who has been hypnotized cannot testify in court about anything remembered during or after hypnosis. Consequently, if I consent to hypnosis, there is a possibility that anything I remember once the hypnosis begins will not be admissible in a court of law. The only way to fully protect my potential right to testify is to forgo the use of hypnosis.

Release from Liability. I understand that, because of the rulings of some legal authorities, there may be limitations placed on my ability to rely on recollections after hypnosis for the purposes of litigation. For example, there is a possibility that anything I remember once hypnosis begins may not be admissible in a court of law. I acknowledge that (therapist's name) has advised me that if I have any concerns about the legal consequences of hypnosis, that I should consult with my own attorney prior to the use of hypnosis. I hereby agree, freely and voluntarily, to undergo hypnosis. I further agree to release and hold harmless (therapist's name) from any claims or liabilities arising from the use of or inability to use my recollections, the therapist's notes, audiotapes or videotapes of therapy sessions, or any other limitations on my or the therapist's testimony in a courtroom or forensic setting. In consenting to hypnosis, I hereby agree that I do not have a cause of action against (therapist's name) based on his/her professional and competent use of hypnosis with me.

Signed _____

Date _____

American Society of Clinical Hypnosis (ASCH) Code of Conduct

Introduction

The ASCH Code of Conduct is comprised of two sections, Ethical Principles and Ethical Standards. The Ethical Principles serve as philosophical guidelines that help to structure a member's practice of hypnosis. The Ethical Standards serve as practical or applied guidelines for the member's practice.

Acceptance of membership in, or Certification by, ASCH commits the member or certified clinician to the Code of Conduct. For the purposes of this document, both ASCH members and those non-members certified by ASCH will be referred to as "members."

In subscribing to this Code, members are required to cooperate in its implementation and abide by any disciplinary rulings based upon this Code. Members should take adequate measures to discourage, prevent, expose, and correct unethical conduct of colleagues. Additionally, members should be equally available to defend and assist colleagues unjustly charged with unethical conduct.

The Code should not be used as an instrument to deprive any member of the opportunity or freedom to practice with complete professional integrity; nor should any disciplinary action be taken on the basis of this Code without maximum provision for safeguarding the rights of the member(s) affected.

Ethical Principles

I. Competence: Members strive to attain the highest levels of professional competence.
   A. Members use hypnosis only within the bounds of their training and expertise; within their primary discipline; and within the context of a professional relationship;
      1. A "professional relationship" is defined by the member's primary discipline and includes consultation or supervision of colleagues.
   B. Members' expertise is determined, in part, by their professional education, training, licensure, and experience;
   C. Members recognize, and are respectful of, any limitations to their expertise;
   D. Members strive to maintain current knowledge of research, issues, and methods in hypnosis;
      1. Members participate in continuing education activities.
II. Professional Responsibility: Members serve the best interests of their clients or patients.
   A. Members accept responsibility for the care of their clients or patients consistent with their discipline and licensure;
   B. Members seek out consultation and/or supervision when in doubt regarding their clinical practices or when questioned by others about their clinical practice;
   C. Members participate and cooperate with inquiries regarding their practice;
   D. Members accept responsibility for, and when necessary the consequences of, their behavior;
   E. Members accept responsibility to monitor and make appropriate changes in their practice to comply with the Ethical Principles or Ethical Standards of this Code;
   F. Members seek to educate the public about the proper and scientific use of hypnosis.

Ethical Standards

I. ASCH members uphold the professional standards, ethics, and codes of conduct of their primary discipline.

II. ASCH members remain in good standing in the association or society that oversees the member's primary discipline.

III. ASCH members maintain a license to practice at the independent, unrestricted, or unsupervised level.

IV. ASCH members do not support the practice of hypnosis by laypersons.

   A. The "practice of hypnosis" means the provision of services, or the offer to provide services, utilizing hypnosis to individuals or groups, regardless if a fee or honorarium is charged, offered, or paid.

   B. A "layperson" is:

      1. an individual lacking professional education and clinical training in a health care discipline, including but not limited to those recognized by ASCH for membership and/or certification,

      or

      2. an individual not pursuing a degree, from a regionally accredited institution, in a health care discipline including but limited to those recognized by ASCH for membership and/or certification.

   C. Members do not provide hypnosis training to laypersons.

V. Public and Media Presentation

   A. ASCH members do not use hypnosis for entertainment purposes.

   B. When members do appear in public forums, such as on television or some other audio or video format, they take care to ensure that any demonstration of hypnosis is done in such a way as to prevent or minimize risk to unknown audience participants.

      1. For example, when a videotape demonstration is shown on television, the member takes steps to ensure that the complete audio portion of the induction and deepening phases are muted.

   C. ASCH members ensure when they present hypnosis, in any format, to the public the member does so within the spirit of this Code and within the guidelines of their primary discipline.

   D. Members honestly and fairly represent their professional competency, qualifications, and capabilities to the public and media, and refrain from making false, misleading, deceptive, or unsubstantiated statements in resumes, advertising, and other means of soliciting clients or patients.

VI. Nothing in this Code shall prohibit members from:

A. teaching hypnosis to individuals or groups who, upon completion of such training, would be eligible for ASCH membership,

B. teaching students of healthcare disciplines, including but not limited to those recognized by ASCH for membership and/or certification,

C. teaching patients or clients the use of self-hypnosis for that individual's own therapeutic use, or

D. teaching about hypnosis in any forum that serves to properly educate and inform the consumer or professional public about hypnosis.

VII. When ASCH members engage in human subjects research, they do so within the accepted standards of their primary discipline, taking precautions not to cause emotional or physical harm to their subjects.

VIII. When this Code is unclear on an issue, question, or complaint and when deemed appropriate by the ASCH Executive Committee, guidance is sought from the ethical standards of the member's primary discipline professional association and/or the member's licensing board.

Enforcement

I. Any person, whether or not a member of ASCH, may initiate a charge of ethical violation against a member of ASCH.

II. Any charge must be submitted in writing to the Ethics Committee, must specify the time and place of the violation, and must be signed by the complainant.

III. The Ethics Committee shall inform the member in writing of the charges against the member and solicit the member's response to the charges.

IV. If, upon receiving the response of the member, the Ethics Committee determines that cause for further inquiry exists, the Ethics Committee shall set a time and place for a hearing and shall notify the member and the complainant, by certified mail, of the time and place.

V. The purpose of the Ethics Committee hearing is to gather all the facts related to the alleged violation. The charged member shall have the privilege of appearing in person, or may submit a written defense to the Ethics Committee at least twenty-four hours prior to the time of the hearing. At the hearing, the charged member shall have the right to cross-examine the complainant and any witnesses who may appear against the member. The charged member shall also have the right to present witnesses. The complainant shall be able to direct questions to the charged member only through a committee member. The hearing may be recorded and a transcript of the proceedings, if any, shall be available at cost.

VI. No later than thirty days following the hearing, the Ethics Committee shall submit a report of its findings to the Executive Committee and recommend either:

A. dismissal of the charges,

B. censure or warning,

C. suspension, or

D. expulsion.

The Ethics Committee shall send by certified mail a copy of its report and recommendation to the charged member.

VII. If the Ethics Committee finds for a recommendation of guilt of any of the charges or recommends censure, warning, suspension, or expulsion, the member shall have thirty days from the receipt of the Ethics Committee report to submit to the Executive Committee written objections to the findings or recommendations of the Ethics Committee.

VIII. The Executive Committee shall review the findings and recommendation of the Ethics Committee and any written objections submitted by the member and shall reach a final decision. In accordance with the By-Laws, the Executive Committee shall not expel a member without holding a hearing at which the accused may appear and be represented by counsel. The Executive Committee shall also have the right to be represented by counsel at such a hearing. The Executive Committee shall notify the member in writing, by certified mail, of its decision.

IX. In accordance with the By-Laws, a decision of censure or warning will be a matter of Executive Committee record only. A decision of suspension or expulsion will be reported to the Board of Governors and to the membership of ASCH through the *Corrections to the Directory* section of the Newsletter.

Approved
4/6/2003

Index

A

Abuse
  childhood, 54, 115
  emotional, 5
  sexual, 5
Adolescent, oppositional behavior, 50
Adult attention deficit disorder, 29
African-American spirituals, 104
Age
  progression, 56, 60, 71, 123
  regression, 54, 55, 80, 102
American Psychological Association (APA),·
  15
  Code, 16
  Ethical Principles of Psychologists, 15
American Society of Clinical Hypnosis
  (ASCH), 16, 141, 147
  Annual Meetings, 20
  Code of Conduct, 147–151
    enforcement, 150–151
    ethical principles, 148
    ethical standards, 149–150
  Committee on Hypnosis and Memory,
    24
Amnesia, 107
  definition of, 57
  partial, 63
Anesthesia, 107
  definition of, 56
  glove, 63
Anger, 50, 108
Anxiety, 105
  beliefs and, 127
  disorder, 95
  hypnotic phenomena and treatment of,
    125
  mental cyclone and, 29

performance, 9, 90
symptoms
  hypnotic phenomena and, 121
  self-hypnosis and, 14
trance and, 12
use of relaxation skills to control, 126
APA, *see* American Psychological
  Association
Apposition of opposites, 54
Arm
  drop technique, Chaisson, 125
  levitation, 58, 71
ASCH, *see* American Society of Clinical
  Hypnosis
Association, 57
Attachments, definition of, 113
Auditory sensory system, 42

B

Behavioral goal setting, 2
Behavioral therapist, 5
Belief system filter, 4
Bodily process, observation of, 75
Body language, 40
Breathing pattern, 82
Brief therapy, 4

C

Catalepsy, 60, 80
  common way of inducing, 58
  emotional, 110
Chaisson, 71, 125
Childhood
  abuse, 54, 115
  identity, 129